THE AUTOIMMUNE PALEO COOKBOOK

AN ALLERGEN-FREE APPROACH TO MANAGING CHRONIC ILLNESS

BY MICKEY TRESCOTT, NTP

Fourth Printing, 2014

Printed in South Korea

ISBN: 978-0-578-13521-2

Library of Congress Control Number: 2013922585

The Autoimmune Paleo Cookbook can be purchased at discount in bulk. Please contact:

Trescott LLC
P.O. Box 20382
Seattle, WA 98102
(503) 487-0044
autoimmunepaleo@gmail.com

Photography: Kyle Johnson, www.kjphotos.com
Styling: Brenna Rose Designs, www.brennarosedesigns.com
Design: Chris Black, www.theblackresidence.com
Cover Design: Chris Black and Kimberly Myers
Copyediting: Lisa Gordanier, www.hiddenhandediting.com

Disclaimer:

The content presented in this book is meant for inspiration and informational purposes only. The purchaser of this book understands that the author is not a medical professional, and the information contained within this book is not intended to replace medical advice or meant to be relied upon to treat, cure, or prevent any disease, illness, or medical condition. It is understood that you will seek full medical clearance by a licensed physician before making any changes mentioned in this book. The author and publisher claim no responsibility to any person or entity for any liability, loss, or damage caused or alleged to be caused directly or indirectly as a result of the use, application, or interpretation of the material in this book.

Dedication:

I would like to dedicate this book to those with chronic illness who are looking to bring healing into their lives.

I would also like to dedicate this book to my sister Katie, for being a constant force of youthful energy and support in my life.

FOREWORD

Diet and lifestyle modifications can be extraordinarily powerful strategies to regulate the immune system, reverse chronic disease, heal the body, and promote overall health. I have a very thorough understanding of the nitty gritty details of how compounds in our foods, the nutrient density of our diets, our hormones, and the 70 trillion probiotic bacteria that live in our guts all interact with our immune system. And I have personal experience with using diet and lifestyle to successfully manage and reverse immune and autoimmune disorders. But I also know that, as powerful as the diet and lifestyle recommendations of The Paleo Approach are, it can also be overwhelming!

Seeing dramatic improvement in your health can be a great motivator to stick to a restricted diet, but that still doesn't mean that it's easy. And for many, just looking at a list of food "don'ts" can stimulate the fight-or-flight response. The initial reaction usually includes a mix of panic and trepidation as well as a flood of questions: "What is there left to eat?" "How can I possibly make yummy food with such limited ingredients?" "How will I survive without my favorite comfort foods or convenience foods?" "How on earth will I entertain company without feeding them bland, weird foods?" And sometimes, we can feel like it's going just fine until we see someone enjoying a piece of cake and then the sense of deprivation hits us like a ton of bricks.

But you don't need to be intimidated by making big changes to your diet and you don't need to miss out on flavor because The Autoimmune Paleo Cookbook has you covered. Simple summary of "the rules"? Check. Strategies for day-to-day implementation? Check. Meal plans and shopping lists? Check. Amazingly delicious recipes? Check and check!

Mickey Trescott is one of the most talented and creative chefs I know. Her recipes combine flavors in a sophisticated yet simple way, using standard cooking techniques and equipment so that anyone can make them. This book includes a variety of palate-pleasing recipes that comply with the recommendations in The Paleo Approach, including: quick everyday meals, elaborate and decadent meals that you could serve to company (and they will never know that they're eating foods belonging to a restricted diet), comfort foods, appetizers, snacks, quick lunches, and luscious desserts.

The most important contribution that The AutoimmunePaleo Cookbook will make to your life is to reintroduce deliciousness! Being able to eat scrumptious, comforting foods and even enjoy the occasional dessert stops that feeling of "missing out" in its tracks. It gives you back the contribution that yummy food makes to your quality of life (while also improving your quality of life via a nutritional upgrade). Yes, you can still enjoy good food even while you eat to regulate your immune system and heal your body.

The Autoimmune Paleo Cookbook also helps you get organized with its resources, guides, tips and tricks, meal plans and shopping lists. This takes the guesswork out of what to eat and helps you plan for the week ahead, a strategy that can be essential for success. As much as this cookbook caters to those who follow the Paleo Approach to manage immune and autoimmune conditions, this is just plain ol' good food. This book could grace any kitchen bookshelf and the recipes herein could be enjoyed by anyone. And regardless of the reasons you've picked up this book, you will find yourself coming back to these recipes over and over again. So grab a fork and get ready to dig in!

Dr. Sarah Ballantyne, PhD, author of The Paleo Approach

INTRODUCTION

What inspired you to pick up this cookbook? Well, like 50 million other Americans, you may have been diagnosed with an autoimmune disease, a condition that occurs when the immune system mistakenly attacks one's own tissue.[1] Given that conventional medicine has yet to find a cause or a cure for this condition, you may be left wondering if there is anything you can do to help yourself. Ask your doctor, and you will likely be told that what you eat has nothing to do with your symptoms. However, if you look at how our modern diet has evolved in the last century, with a marked increase in the over-processing of many foods and the emphasis on grains, refined sugar, chemicals, toxins, and pesticides, among other elements, it's hard not to see that the food we choose to put into our bodies every day has a direct impact on the rapid increase in chronic illness. What we eat does matter, and just as an improper diet can cause disease, a nourishing one can bring healing—even with a condition as serious as autoimmune disease.

This book is the product of my own personal struggle to find health and vitality using the Autoimmune Protocol—a version of an ancestral diet that removes foods such as grains, beans, dairy, eggs, nuts, seeds, and nightshades (a family of plants containing foods like tomatoes, potatoes, eggplant, and peppers). This diet is designed to heal the gut, or more specifically, the small intestine, which scientists have now pinpointed as a major factor contributing to autoimmune disease.[2]

It was only a short time ago that I felt lost in my own health struggle, not knowing which foods were safe for me to consume or what I could do to manage my condition. I knew I was having food reactions, but I didn't know exactly which foods were causing them. You can imagine then, the excitement I felt after discovering the Autoimmune Protocol and starting to see changes for the better–I finally felt like I had my life back! I used this new found energy to get back into the kitchen to develop recipes that were free from ingredients that would trigger my symptoms.

In this book I have taken everything I learned on my journey back to health and packaged it so that you can re-create this process for yourself. Implementing the Autoimmune Protocol will help you pinpoint your food allergies and sensitivities as well as gauge how they are affecting your disease. By using this method, you'll find a diet that is most supportive of your individual healing process.

In the first half of the book, you will find a description of exactly what the protocol is, charts of what to eat and what to avoid, which foods you can include to promote healing, as well as meal plans and shopping lists to help you transition more quickly. If you're a little more cautious or need more time, I encourage you to start incorporating some of the meals into your routine little by little. Although completely eliminating the problematic foods will have the quickest effect, any move toward a cleaner, more allergen-free diet will help you in the long run.

If there is one takeaway from this book, it is that you do not have to suffer eating a bland, boring diet while eliminating potential food triggers and attempting to regain your health. Despite how daunting it may sound on paper, it is entirely possible to eat varied, flavorful, and interesting meals while on the Autoimmune Protocol, even if some of the most common and convenient foods are removed. Many of these recipes are simple, delicious versions of familiar

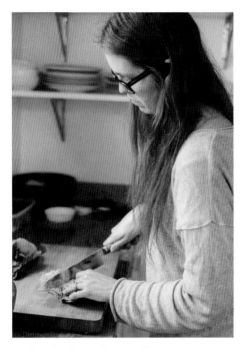

dishes—like "Spaghetti" and Meatballs (page 282), Chicken Caesar Salad (page 154), or Clam Chowder (page 254). I've also included recipes with ingredients that are a little more out of the ordinary for those who wish to try new flavors, like Moroccan Lamb Stew (page 174), Coconut-Basil Pesto (page 124), Orange-Rosemary Duck (page 220), or Mushroom-Stuffed Cornish Hens (page 223). Armed with these recipes, you can easily create a menu that dinner-party guests will be thrilled to share. Don't be surprised at holiday meals when your allergen-free desserts are consumed more quickly than the conventional ones!

Another thing to be aware of: eating this way is never going to be as easy as eating a standard American diet. It takes a lot of discipline, energy, and time to successfully make the switch. Even after the transition is made, there will still be an unusual amount of planning and organization required to keep your kitchen stocked with healing foods at all times. Once you get into a routine, though, tasks like making Solid Cooking Fat (page 42), Fermented Vegetables (page 37), and Bone Broth (page 34), and keeping your freezer stocked full of pastured meats and emergency meals becomes easier. Your kitchen starts to have an ebb and flow; one day you bottle kombucha and roast a chicken, the next you make some broth with the bones. While in the beginning you may need to follow a strict plan and commit everything to paper, you might be surprised when you no longer have to obsess over the details; maintaining the diet becomes routine.

If you are anything like I was at the time I discovered the Autoimmune Protocol, you may be in poor health and without ample time or energy to cook. For those in this circumstance, I've done my best to include simple, one-pot meals that can be prepared ahead and used when you need a quick meal. Most of the soups, like Beet and Fennel Soup (page 157), Carrot-Ginger Soup (page 157), Classic Chicken Soup (page 160), and Under the Weather Soup (page 172) can be cooked as a double batch and frozen in portion-size containers. Shredded Chicken Breast (page 208) and Shredded Roast Beef (page 256) can be also be cooked in quantity and used to create tasty meals during the week. If you can, recruit willing friends and family members to help you keep healthy food on hand. Once you regain some of your strength and energy, you'll be able to branch out into recipes that require more preparation.

Lastly, on page 302 you will find a section devoted to resources helpful to anyone searching for more information on diet and autoimmunity. There are books and websites on ancestral nutrition, autoimmune disease, and digestion that make an excellent supplement to the information presented here. I have also included links to resources for finding pastured meat in your area, as well as sources for finding practitioners who can help guide you on your path to better health.

MY STORY

In my mid-twenties, following the investigation of some growing health concerns, I was diagnosed with two conditions: Hashimoto's disease (an autoimmune disease that targets the thyroid gland) and Celiac disease (an autoimmune disease that targets the small intestine). Prior to this experience, I barely knew what an autoimmune disease was, and only knew of a friend-of-a-friend who had one. While I had previously been an active, healthy person, my condition declined rather quickly, until I was unable to work or do any of the activities that I had previously loved—like cycling, rock climbing, and running. I sought the help of both conventional and alternative medicine, neither of which had any effective options for me. After months of resting, waiting, and further testing, I still didn't have any answers. It was then that I embarked on my own search for healing.

I have always been a believer in food as medicine. Ten years prior, while in college, I experimented with veganism, which resulted in many initial health benefits—the best of which was the disappearance of my severe asthma. I later found out that this condition stemmed from a serious dairy allergy that had been misdiagnosed as asthma in childhood. It was then that I learned how to cook, and I eliminated all processed foods from my diet. While I felt great when I first adopted this diet, after a couple of years I started having some new health concerns: low energy, hair loss, and fatigue. When I went to the doctor, I discovered that I was suffering from vitamin deficiencies and would need to rely on supplements to keep my levels up. I thought that these vitamins were all I needed to keep me healthy, but over the years I noticed a steady decline in my energy level and overall health.

By the time I was diagnosed with my autoimmune conditions, I was struggling to get through each day, and relying heavily on caffeine and sugar. After my crash, I asked all of the doctors I saw what they thought of my vegan diet—I wanted to know if it could be one of the reasons I wasn't recovering. They reassured me that a low-fat, plant-based diet with proper supplementation was excellent for my condition. Despite their advice, I was getting worse with every passing month. I tried raw food diets and more supplements, as well as cleanses, some of which further weakened my condition and made me more ill.

In an act of desperation, I decided to entertain the thought that maybe the way I was eating was not optimal for my body. It was from this place that I began to research the connection between diet and autoimmune disease. Through testimonials of those who had healed from chronic health issues, I discovered the concept of the ancestral, or Paleo, style of eating. What I found was the notion that a nourishing diet that included the foods of our ancestors and excluded modern convenience products was ideal for maximum healing. I immediately cut out the grains and beans I had been living off of, and slowly started introducing pastured meats, eggs, and wild-caught fish into my diet. I started eating organ meats like liver and soups made with bone broth. After making these changes, I was quickly relieved of the worst of my coldness and fatigue. This encouraged me to believe I was on the right track, although I knew there were still some foods in my diet holding me back from restoring my health.

As I continued my research, I found the work of Dr. Datis Kharrazian, who advocates for a specific diet to heal the gut for those with autoimmune disease.[3] Around the same time, I also discovered that many of the leaders in the ancestral health movement, like Robb Wolf, were advocating a similar approach called the Autoimmune Protocol.[4] All of these experts were basing their recommendations on research in the scientific literature that linked autoimmune disease to gut health. It was apparent that there were additional foods that could be problematic for those with autoimmune disease. This made sense to me, as I had found some success with my diet change but knew that I was still having trouble with certain foods—it was just a matter of pinpointing which ones. All of these sources were leading me in the direction of trying an elimination diet to find out which specific foods I was sensitive to.

I decided to try the Autoimmune Protocol for a few months. Initially, it did not go well. I was tortured by how few foods I could have, and I did not experience the immediate benefits that I had heard of others experiencing. After a few failed starts, I managed to stick with it, and after a few months I felt a shift in my energy. I attempted to reintroduce foods, and my efforts were met with a crashing return of symptoms. It was here that I decided to commit to the Autoimmune Protocol long-term, and I continued to see benefits with every passing month. I also started to dig deeper into making lifestyle changes in order to be more gentle on myself and give my body the rest it needed to heal. After another few months of sticking to my plan, I was my healthy, vibrant self once again.

Although it was not the only factor that contributed to my recovery, finding the Autoimmune Protocol and eliminating my food triggers was an incredibly powerful piece of the healing journey. Along with changing my diet, I enlisted the help of a functional medicine practitioner—a doctor who specializes in treating patients as a whole, from a perspective of health instead of disease. I also made the lifestyle modifications recommended by those in the ancestral health community—mainly stress management, sleep, and movement. In order to be successful, I believe a multi-faceted approach such as this gives the best results.

It has been years since my original transition to the Autoimmune Protocol, and although I have been able to incorporate many of the "foods to avoid" into my diet on a somewhat regular basis, I always return to the stricter protocol in periods of illness or stress. At one point, I struggled with feeling sorry for myself because I realized that I wouldn't be eating certain foods ever again, and would always mistrust the food prepared at restaurants. Now, if anything, I am overjoyed that I found out what works for me, and I am constantly thinking of new ways to prepare safe foods that are creative and flavorful, and that I can share with those I love. Instead of eating out, I enjoy cooking and collaborating with my friends, both those with food allergies and without. Even though this has been a long road, I am forever grateful for the ability to learn how certain foods negatively affect my body, and how other foods bring nourishment and vitality into my life.

THE AUTOIMMUNE
PROTOCOL

ANCESTRAL DIETS EXPLAINED

Before delving into the specifics of the dietary modifications that help those of us with autoimmune disease, I must explain the ancestral health movement. In the last few years there have been a growing number of health experts, doctors, and researchers advocating a new way of eating in order to address the growing health concerns of our modern society—and their answer, in a nutshell, is to eat like our ancestors. How that is defined exactly is up to each advocate and their respective followers, but they all agree that modern foods like grains, beans, refined sugar, vegetable oils, and food chemicals are out. In addition to excluding these modern foods, there is also emphasis on adding high-quality animal foods that were available to our ancestors: pastured meats, wild-caught fish, as well as making use of the "odd bits" like bones and organ meats.[5]

Through eating this way, a growing number of people have found a path to better health and vitality, whether it be better sleep, weight loss, improved digestion, mood, or increased energy. Some of the most compelling stories coming out of this movement are the reports of those who suffered for years with chronic health issues that have now been resolved. When the body is given whole, natural foods, free from processing, chemicals, and toxins, it enables the natural processes we all have within us to detoxify and heal.

WHAT IS THE AUTOIMMUNE PROTOCOL?

Although eating like our ancestors can be quite powerful at reversing a number of health conditions, it has been recommended by experts in the community that those with autoimmune diseases make further restrictions, at least until the condition is put into remission. The Autoimmune Protocol, also known as the Paleo Approach, is the variation that has been recommended for those with autoimmune conditions.[6] While most ancestral diets avoid grains, beans, legumes, and dairy, the Autoimmune Protocol also removes eggs, nuts, seeds, and nightshade vegetables (such as tomatoes and peppers—more on that later), food chemicals (like thickeners and alternative sweeteners), and over-the-counter medications like NSAIDs (such as ibuprofen). In addition to removing of all of these products, there is an emphasis placed on replacing them with the highest quality, most nutrient-dense foods available: pastured meats, wild-caught fish, organ meats, bone broth, fermented foods, and a colorful array of fruits and vegetables.[7]

Sarah Ballantyne, author of *The Paleo Approach*, has done the most thorough research on the subject, and this book follows her version of the protocol. In addition to dietary modifications, there are many important lifestyle changes that are integral to healing from autoimmune disease that are covered in Sarah's book—increasing sleep, lessening stress, increasing movement, and optimizing sun exposure.

WHY DOES IT WORK?

The main premise of the Autoimmune Protocol is that it is designed to help heal the gut from both intestinal permeability (otherwise known as "leaky gut") as well as dysbiosis, both of which have been shown to be present in those with autoimmune disease.[8] Leaky gut occurs when the tight junctions of the cells lining the small intestine become more permeable, letting undigested food, toxins, and pathogens into the body, triggering the immune system.[9] Dysbiosis is an imbalance of gut flora (the microorganisms that live in the digestive tract), leading to overgrowths or deficiencies of certain species.[10] Research has shown that the foods and substances avoided on the Autoimmune Protocol contribute to both of these conditions. By removing them from the diet, the gut lining is then able to heal, and proper flora balance can be established. This almost always results in a lessening of symptoms and healing for those facing autoimmune disease.[11]

FOODS TO AVOID

GRAINS

amaranth
barley
buckwheat
bulgur
corn
farro
kamut
millet
oats
quinoa
rice
rye
sorghum
spelt
teff
triticale
wheat
wild rice

NUTS

almond
brazil
cashew
coffee
cocoa
hazelnut
pecan
pine nut
pistachio
macadamia
walnut

BEANS + LEGUMES

adzuki beans
black beans
black-eyed peas
broad beans
chickpeas
fava beans
garbanzo beans
kidney beans
lentils
lima beans
mung beans
navy beans
peanuts
red beans
soybeans
white beans

SEEDS

anise
canola
caraway
chia
coriander
cumin
fennel seed
fennugreek
flax
mustard
nutmeg
poppy
pumpkin
sesame
sunflower
hemp

EGGS

chicken eggs
duck eggs
goose eggs
quail eggs

DAIRY

butter
buttermilk
casein
cheese
condensed milk
cottage cheese
cream
cream cheese
evaporated milk
frozen yogurt
goat cheese
goat milk
ice cream
ghee
kefir
milk
powdered milk
sheep milk
sour cream
whey
whey protein
whipped cream
yogurt

NIGHTSHADES

cayenne pepper
chili pepper
chipotle chili pepper
eggplant
goji berry
ground cherry
habanero pepper
jalepeño pepper
paprika
poblano pepper
potato
sweet pepper
tobacco
tomato
tomatillo
wolf berries

OTHER

alcohol
alternative sweeteners
emulsifiers
food additives
food chemicals
NSAIDs (aspirin,
   ibuprofen, naproxen)
stevia
thickeners

FOODS TO INCLUDE

VEGETABLES

artichoke
arugula
asparagus
bok choi
broccoli
brussels sprouts
butternut squash
cabbage
cauliflower
celery
chard
collard green
cucumber
fennel
kale
leek
lettuce
mushroom
pumpkin
rhubarb
snap pea
spinach
summer squash
watercress
winter squash
zucchini

FATS

animal fat
avocado oil
coconut oil
duck fat
lard
olive oil
palm oil
tallow

ROOTS

beet
carrot
celeriac
jicama
onion
parsnip
turnip
radish
rutabaga
shallot
sweet potato
yam

MEATS

beef
bison
buffalo
lamb
fish
shellfish
chicken
turkey
duck
pork
rabbit
venison

OFFAL

bone broth
gizzard
heart
kidney
liver
tongue

FRUIT

apple
apricot
avocado
banana
blackberry
blueberry
cantaloupe
cherry
clementine
coconut
date
fig
grape
grapefruit
guava
huckleberry
honeydew
kiwi
lemon
lime
mango
marionberry
nectarine
orange
papaya
peach
pear
persimmon
plum
pineapple
pomegranate
raspberry
strawberry
tangerine
watermelon

HERBS

basil
bay leaves
chamomile
chives
cilantro
dill
lavender
lemongrass
marjoram
mint
parsley
peppermint
rosemary
sage
spearmint
tarragon
thyme

SPICES

cinnamon
cloves
garlic
ginger
saffron
sea salt
shallots
tea
turmeric

PANTRY

apple cider vinegar
anchovies
arrowroot powder
coconut flour
coconut flakes
coconut vinegar
coconut aminos
olives
oysters
salmon
sardines
tuna
ume plum vinegar

OCCASIONAL SWEETENERS

dates
dried fruit
honey
maple syrup
molasses

FERMENTS

sauerkraut
fermented vegetables
    (carrots, beets,
    other vegetables)
kombucha
water kefir

THE ARGUMENT FOR NUTRIENT DENSITY

While avoiding foods that contribute to leaky gut and dysbiosis are an important part of the protocol, equally important is increasing the amount of nutrient-dense foods. These nutrients are desperately needed by the body to heal the gut and nourish the body. It may seem like the elimination of so many foods from the diet would result in nutrient deficiencies, but that is hardly the case—this way of eating is much more nutrient-dense than the standard American diet and is perfectly healthy to continue long-term. It is particularly high in nutrients needed for healing and recovery: the fat-soluble vitamins A and D, the B vitamins, omega-3 fatty acids, as well as other minerals and nutrients like zinc, selenium, carotenoids, and sulfur. Given this, in order to be successful you must diligently seek out the most nutrient-dense foods and include them in your diet on a regular basis.

This means eating a varied diet that includes organ meats like liver and kidney, fatty fish and shellfish, seaweed, fermented foods, and tons of colorful fruits and vegetables. Do not ignore this piece of the protocol! A lot of these foods are not common or palatable for many, but they were an integral part of our ancestors' diets. I would encourage you to step out of your comfort zone and make an effort to include these foods in order to bring more of these nutrients into your diet.

Here is a list of important nutrients and some of the Autoimmune Protocol compliant foods they are found in.[12] This list is by no means exhaustive, but you can see why it is of the utmost importance to include certain foods in your diet (dare I mention liver and fatty fish?):

FAT-SOLUBLE VITAMINS

Vitamin A: Liver and fish liver oil (for retinol), yellow-orange vegetables (for beta carotene, which is a precursor to vitamin A)

Vitamin D: Liver and fish liver oil, fatty fish, and sunlight exposure

Vitamin E: Red palm oil, coconut oil, olive oil, green leafy vegetables

Vitamin K: Organ meats, cruciferous and dark green leafy vegetables, fermented foods

OTHER NUTRIENTS

Carotenoids: Colorful vegetables (like carrots, squash, sweet potatoes, and beets)

Essential Fatty Acids: Fatty fish and fish liver oil, pastured meats, organ meats

Sulfur: Cruciferous vegetables (broccoli, kale, cabbage)

WATER-SOLUBLE VITAMINS

B vitamins: Meat and seafood (especially shellfish and organ meats), colorful vegetables, seaweed

Vitamin C: Colorful fruits and vegetables, especially citrus and green leafy vegetables

MINERALS

Calcium: Dark green leafy vegetables, bone broth, sardines

Copper: Shellfish, liver

Iodine: Fish, shellfish, seaweed

Iron: Muscle meat, organ meat, fish, shellfish, dark green leafy vegetables

Magnesium: Dark green leafy vegetables, orange vegetables, bone broth, sardines

Potassium: Fish, cruciferous and dark green leafy vegetables, orange vegetables

Selenium: Fish, shellfish, organ meats, muscle meats

Zinc: Shellfish, organ meats, muscle meats, green leafy vegetables

OTHER FACTORS

In addition to removing specific foods and increasing the overall nutrient density of your diet, there are other factors that can help you on your road to recovery. Although this book is mostly about the dietary aspect of healing, it would be incomplete without the acknowledgement of some of the lifestyle factors that are crucial for recovering your health. For more information about these and other steps you can take to help yourself through this process, I highly recommend checking out Sarah Ballantyne's incredible book, *The Paleo Approach*, where she goes into more detail about these important lifestyle changes.

· **Sleep:** Make sure you are sleeping well—this is essential for healing and allowing your body to restore itself. Aim for at least eight hours uninterrupted sleep per night—more if you can manage it.

· **Stress Management:** Engage in at least one activity aimed at reducing your stress level every day, whether it be meditation, walking, taking a bath, or anything else that helps you relax.

· **Movement:** Make an effort to do one movement-based activity every day. This could be gentle exercise like yoga, qigong, or walking, or a more intense activity like bike riding, running or hiking.

· **Sunlight exposure:** It is very important to get sunlight exposure on some part of your body (it could just be your face and arms) for 20 minutes every day. This stimulates your body's production of vitamin D, which is extremely important to the healing process.

In addition to these lifestyle factors, finding a practitioner trained in functional medicine can be an invaluable part of monitoring your progress with testing as well as making individual supplement recommendations. Be sure to visit the resources section (page 302) as well as my website to find practitioners who integrate dietary approaches into their practices.

REINTRODUCING FOODS

At some point after implementing the Autoimmune Protocol, a person should start to see improvement (and in some cases even remission). This usually takes at least a month, but can take up to a few months or more of eating strictly according to the protocol. Once a person starts to see a measurable improvement, it is up to them whether they want to play it safe and continue on (in an effort to experience deeper healing), or if they want to try to reintroduce some of the "safer," disallowed foods. The point at which a person arrives at the place where reintroductions are possible is highly individual, and there is no way to tell how long it will be until you try.

That being said, it is extremely important *not* to start reintroducing foods until you see a *measurable* improvement in your symptoms. If you start too soon, you will have nothing to gauge your reaction against. I encourage you to stay on the Autoimmune Protocol as long as you can, letting yourself heal as much as possible before reintroducing foods. When it comes time for reintroductions, it will be absolutely clear which foods are affecting you. If you've been on the Autoimmune Protocol for a few months with no improvements, it may be appropriate to enlist the assistance of a functional medicine practitioner to help with further testing. Check the resources on page 302 to help you find one.

The protocol for reintroductions, as outlined by Sarah Ballantyne in *The Paleo Approach*, is the following:

1. Pick a food to challenge and get ready to eat it a couple of times in one day.

2. Eat the food for the first time, only having a nibble. Wait fifteen minutes, and if you don't have any symptoms, take a small bite, a little larger than the last.

3. Wait another fifteen minutes, and if you still don't have any symptoms, take another bite, again slightly larger.

4. Wait two to three hours, watching to see if any symptoms appear.

5. Next, eat an average quantity of the food, either by itself of as a part of a meal.

6. Watch your symptoms for three to seven days afterwards, being sure to avoid the food you reintroduced as well as not reintroducing any other foods.

7. You may incorporate the food into your diet if you have no symptoms during this whole process.

When you reintroduce a food, you are looking for *any* type of reaction to that food. It could be the return or worsening of your autoimmune symptoms: digestive changes or upset, headaches, dizziness, problems with energy or sleep, joint or muscle pain, skin changes like rashes or acne, or even changes in mood. Reactions can be immediate, or they could show up a day or two after the fact. If you think your reaction to a certain food is a coincidence with some other external factor, like illness or stress, wait until you recover and reintroduce again.

I like to keep a journal for tracking food reintroductions. The more information you are able to track, the better. It's a good idea to plan your reintroductions for a time when you are feeling good and not under a lot of stress. This way you have more energy to devote to assessing your condition and tracking the process, and you will know that the symptoms you are experiencing are from the foods and not just from other influences.

According to Sarah Ballantyne, foods should be reintroduced in stages. Those in stage 1 have the highest chance of being tolerated, while those in stage 4 have the least. While you should be careful to only introduce foods one at a time, you should also pay attention to try all of the foods in stage 1 before moving on to stage 2. This means your first food reintroductions should be along the lines of egg yolks and seed spices, not tomatoes or milk (sorry!). Here are the stages, as outlined in *The Paleo Approach*:

STAGE 1:

Egg yolks
Legumes with edible pods
Fruit and berry-based spices
Seed-based spices
Seed and nut oils
Ghee from grass-fed dairy

STAGE 2:

Seeds
Nuts (except cashews and pistachios)
Cocoa or chocolate
Egg whites
Grass-fed butter
Alcohol (in small quantities)

STAGE 3:

Cashews and pistachios
Eggplant
Sweet peppers
Paprika
Coffee
Grass-fed raw cream
Fermented grass-fed raw dairy (yogurt and kefir)

STAGE 4:

Other dairy products (grass-fed whole milk and cheese)
Chili peppers
Tomatoes
Potatoes
Other nightshades and nightshade spices
Alcohol (in larger quantities)
White rice
Traditionally prepared legumes (soaked and fermented)
Traditionally prepared gluten-free grains (soaked and fermented)
Foods you have a history of severe reaction to
Foods you are allergic to

Once you begin reintroducing foods and learning how to gauge your reactions to them, you will start to piece together a safe diet that best manages your condition. While a negative reaction to a food can be discouraging, don't discount that you may be able to tolerate that food a few months down the line as your body continues to heal. My advice is to be cautious, take it slow, and when in doubt, leave it out. Over time, you will learn to better listen to your body's language as it tells you how to discern which foods are promoting health and which ones are slowing your progress.

KITCHEN BASICS

STOCKING YOUR KITCHEN
WITH REAL FOODS

So you've been convinced to try the Autoimmune Protocol with the aim of bringing your body back to health. That is awesome! But how do you convert your kitchen from a place of constant temptation to one that promotes your healing journey?

The first step is to remove all the most obvious foods that will be detrimental to your progress. This means that all items containing gluten, plus processed foods, refined sugar, treats, candy, snack foods, convenience foods, and the like should be removed from your cupboards. If you still have family members who wish to eat these foods, ask them if they would be willing to store them where they won't be encountered in your daily routine (and try to convince them that they shouldn't be eating processed food and sugar anyway!). You do not need to remove everything excluded on the Autoimmune Protocol–things like nuts, seeds, and spices are fine to keep around until you are ready to do reintroductions. It is very important, however, to make sure you get rid of any snacks or quick, easy, convenience foods you could access at a time of weakness during your elimination diet. Examine the ingredients of everything in your cupboards carefully.

Once you have your pantry and cupboards clear, it's time to stock them full of foods you *can* have. While the Autoimmune Protocol lends itself to a lot of fresh cooked food and not a lot to easily storable convenience foods, I have given you some ideas of items you can keep in your pantry that are called for in recipes throughout the book. Other foods, like canned fish, can be useful in case of an emergency when you have no other options available.

Next, you'll want to get into the routine of batch cooking gut-healing foods like Bone Broth (page 34), Fermented Vegetables (page 37), and fermented beverages like Kombucha (page 38) and Water Kefir (page 41). I call for Bone Broth in many of the recipes in this book, and there's a reason for that: it adds gelatin, collagen, minerals, and other nutrients that help heal the gut. It can even replace your morning coffee! Fermented foods and beverages are great to consume in order to get a daily dose of probiotics. While you don't *have* to use these recipes, I believe that incorporating them into your diet gives you the best chance of success while on the Autoimmune Protocol.

In addition to the gut-healing recipes you will learn, having some other basic recipes in your arsenal will make the task of providing yourself nutritious and varied meals a little easier. Rendering your own fat from pastured animals (page 42) is an inexpensive and healthful way to obtain solid cooking fat to use daily in your kitchen. Also, regularly making batches of Coconut Concentrate (page 45) and Creamy Coconut Milk (page 46) cuts down on the time it takes to prepare recipes that call for these ingredients.

Lastly, I have included a section on which kitchen tools you will find useful for preparing the recipes in this book. While you don't need to go out and purchase any wild appliances, there are some basic tools you will need—after all, you'll be spending a lot of time in the kitchen!

PANTRY ITEMS

· Anchovies – Use to flavor dressings and to add to salads. Check the ingredients to ensure they are packed in olive oil and have no other additives—I like the brand Crown Prince.

· Arrowroot starch/flour – I use arrowroot occasionally as a thickener in some of the recipes in this book. Bob's Red Mill sells a large bag of it that is often less expensive than the tiny bottles found in the spice department.

· Avocado oil – A nice oil to have on hand to use in salad dressings and other cold applications. Although I don't call for it in this book, it can replace olive oil in any of the recipes. Purchase a cold-pressed variety, and store it in an opaque bottle away from light and heat, as it oxidizes easily.

· Canned seafood – An excellent choice for emergency meals, especially when you're traveling or on the go. Sardines, salmon, tuna, oysters, and herring are all favorites. Choose brands that are certified for sustainable fishing practices and that pack their products in BPA-free cans. Be sure to double-check the can for avoided ingredients like soybean or cottonseed oil. I like the brands Crown Prince and Wild Planet.

· Coconut aminos – A product made by Leslie's Organics that is similar to soy sauce but is made from coconut. Use in Asian-themed dishes to replace soy sauce. If you have trouble sourcing it, check my online resources (page 304).

· Coconut concentrate (also known as coconut cream, coconut butter, or coconut "manna") – A concentrated coconut flesh product that is solid at room temperature. It can be used to make dressings, thicken sauces and stews, or may be eaten by itself. I have included a recipe to make it (page 45), but it can also be purchased commercially.

· Coconut crystals – Sugar made from the evaporated syrup from coconut trees. I would use this sparingly—I only call for it in one recipe in the book (Apple-Cranberry Crumble, page 299). The brand I like is Leslie's Organics.

· Coconut milk – Use to thicken soups and stews, to add to smoothies, or to drink by itself. The only brand I have found without non-compliant thickeners like guar gum is called Natural Value (Check my online resources, page 304).

· Coconut oil – An excellent solid cooking fat to use for cooking and baking. Look for products that are not processed with heat or chemicals, if possible—I like Tropical Traditions gold label.

· Coconut flour – Flour made from the dried flesh of coconuts. I use this in a couple of the dessert recipes in this book. Again, Leslie's Organics makes an excellent product.

· Dried fruit – Nice to have on hand for the occasional sweet treat or to add to a dessert recipe. I like having dates, raisins, currants, and dried apricots handy.

· Dried herbs and spices – Bay leaves, turmeric, cinnamon, ground ginger, and ground cloves are all seasonings that you should have on hand. If you don't have a source of fresh herbs like thyme, rosemary, sage, oregano, basil, or tarragon, it might be nice to keep a small stock of those in their dried form.

· Gelatin – Although I don't call for it in the book, having some gelatin (from grass-fed animals) is nice if you can't source bones for making broth. It can also be used to thicken desserts and to make gummy candies. I like the brand Great Lakes because it comes from pastured animals.

· Honey – I have this on hand to use sparingly when I need just a touch of sweetness. If possible, choose a raw honey local to your area.

· Maple syrup – I like this ingredient because it adds a complex flavor to desserts, although I would recommend not going overboard with sweeteners while on the protocol. Grade B is preferable because it is richer in nutrients.

· Olives – Olives are a common recipe ingredient and are excellent to have on hand for snacks and to add to salads. Be sure to check the label for ingredients other than oil or vinegar, and avoid purchasing any olives in bulk if you are not sure of the ingredients (many places pack them in seed oils and add nightshade spices).

· Extra-virgin olive oil – An excellent oil for using cold, like adding to already-cooked fish or salad dressings. Choose a high-quality, pure oil (free from additives) that is sold in an opaque bottle. Be sure to store away from light and heat, as it oxidizes easily.

· Sea salt – Sea salt is full of trace minerals and free from anti-caking agents and additives. The type is not as important as its level of processing (least processed is best).

· Tapioca starch/flour – I use tapioca as a thickener in a few of the recipes in this book, but some people with severe gluten intolerance may be sensitive to it—in this case use arrowroot instead.

· Unsweetened coconut flakes – These are dried flakes made from the flesh of fresh coconut. Use them as an addition to salads and to make snacks and desserts. They can also be blended to make your own Coconut Concentrate (page 45). Be sure to purchase the full-fat, unsweetened variety. It's nice to have both large- and small-flake varieties on hand.

· Vinegar – Any type of vinegar is acceptable to use on the Autoimmune Protocol, but the label still must be checked for gluten-free status. Some aged vinegars are stored in casks sealed with wheat paste, so if you have a product in mind, it may be a good idea to call the company just to double check. I like to have apple cider vinegar (Braggs brand) ume plum vinegar (Eden brand) and coconut vinegar (Leslie's Organics brand) on hand.

GUT-HEALING FOODS

Removing certain foods from the diet is only part of the Autoimmune Protocol—in order to be successful, you must also pay careful attention to increasing the nutrient density and incorporating healing foods into your diet. I am a proponent of consuming fermented foods every day, whether that be eating fermented vegetables or having a probiotic beverage like kombucha or water kefir. In addition to ferments, bone broth is an integral part of healing the gut. It can be enjoyed as a warming beverage in the morning or afternoon instead of coffee, and your body will thank you for all of the healing minerals and nutrients contained within. Even if you don't want to drink it by itself, a large majority of the recipes in this book call for it, so it is something you should always have on hand, either fresh or frozen in advance. Please don't replace this with store-bought broth or stock—it is not the same thing. In many cases, commercial broth contains additives and ingredients that are not included on the Autoimmune Protocol, and is not made from pastured, healthfully raised animals.

Bone Broth

Traditionally, humans consumed bone broth as an integral part of soups, stews, and sauces made by using large, bone-in pieces of meat. Over time our culture has strayed from using the whole animal in favor of the leanest cuts of meat, without any trace of the odd bits. This is a travesty considering all of the nutrition that can be gleaned from the leftover bones, cartilage, joints, and marrow we usually throw away. Thankfully, bone broth has been making a comeback due to its many health benefits. Broth is rich in collagen, which is incredibly useful for maintaining healthy joints, skin, and hair, as well as gelatin, which has gut-healing qualities. It is also rich in the minerals that are needed to make bone, which makes it a very restorative and balancing item to include in our diets. Make a batch or two on the weekends and have it available for drinking in the morning instead of coffee, as well as to use in soups, stews, and sauces.

Fermented Vegetables

Many traditional cultures used fermentation as a way to preserve foods for long periods of time without the need for canning or refrigeration. During the process of lacto-fermentation, beneficial bacteria break down the food to make it richer in enzymes and nutrients. These beneficial bacteria promote the growth of healthy gut flora in our intestines and are an integral component of a healing diet. Including a scoop of fermented vegetables every morning with breakfast is a great way to get some of this probiotic food on a regular basis.

Probiotic Beverages

Both kombucha and water kefir are fermented beverages that are made from starter cultures, although they are a little different from each other. Both of them contain probiotics and aid digestion and immune function. While the kombucha contains more acids and enzymes (ideal for aiding digestion), water kefir tends to have more probiotic content. Including one or both is not essential to a gut-healing protocol, but I find them beneficial (and fun to make!).

Kitchen Staples

In addition to some store-bought staples I like to have handy in my pantry, there are a few recipes that I like to make on a weekly basis. Since high-quality, rendered animal fat is both costly and hard to find, I believe it is essential to render your own from fat that you source locally. This is the "solid cooking fat" referenced in many of my recipes, and as you will see from the upcoming section on which fats to cook with, it is essential to do any high-heat cooking with a healthy saturated fat. I also find it preferable to have a couple of different fats available for cooking to add flavor and variety. If you don't have access to quality animal fat in your area, coconut oil and red palm oil are other saturated-fat alternatives.

In addition to having a variety of solid cooking fats to choose from, I like to make a couple of staples from coconut products to have handy for recipes. I call for Coconut Concentrate (page 45) as well as Creamy Coconut Milk (page 46) in many of my recipes to get a creamy consistency. It would be wise to include making these items during your weekly batch-cooking routine so that they can be quickly added to meals and recipes during the week.

BONE BROTH

4 quarts filtered water

2 (or more) pounds bones from a good source (knuckle and marrow bones work well, but you can use any type of bones)

2 tablespoons apple cider vinegar

1 bay leaf

Stovetop method:

1 Place all ingredients in a large stockpot or crock-pot (slow cooker) and bring to a boil. Lower the heat so the water is barely simmering; cover. Occasionally skim the surface for any scum that may appear during cooking.

2 Cook for at least 8 and up to 24 hours, being sure to check periodically to ensure the broth is still at a bare simmer. The longer you cook your bones the more rich and nutritious the broth will be.

Pressure Cooker method:

1 Place all ingredients in a pressure cooker, making sure not to exceed the fill line. Lock the lid and place over high heat until the cooker comes to high pressure, then turn down to the lowest setting that will maintain this pressure (you may need to use a flame tamer).

2 Let the broth cook this way for 3 hours, then turn off the heat and let the broth depressurize and cool naturally.

When the broth is finished (using either method):

3 Let cool, then strain and portion the broth into containers for storage. After the liquid is strained, pick through any bones that are still intact and save them to add to the next batch, tossing those that fell apart. (You can usually get a few batches out of larger beef knuckle bones, while chicken bones last only 1 to 2 batches).

Variation: There are many ways to vary your bone broth, such as browning the bones in the oven before cooking or adding some herbs and spices or vegetables while it is cooking. I like to avoid salting my broth so that it doesn't impact the amount of salt used in recipes. The broth can also be boiled to reduce so that it is concentrated and stored more easily. As you continue to make broth you will get into a flow, and can make it according to your preference. I have added some links to resources on page 304 for further reading on alternate methods as well as the benefits of bone broth.

Sourcing Note: Bones should not be expensive or difficult to find. The best source is from a farmer you trust, maybe at a farmers market or through a CSA. If you don't have those sources available to you, a lot of natural food stores sell bones from grass-fed meat—be sure to ask the butcher if you don't see any available! Also, you can start a bag in your freezer for storing any bones from the meat you consume— just toss them into the bag, and make broth at a later time. Feel free to use any type of bones, even if they have been previously cooked, to make broth—beef, lamb, chicken, and turkey all work well.

Storage: Keeps in the refrigerator for a week. Also freezes well.

SIMPLE SAUERKRAUT

TOOLS	TIME	YIELD	DIFFICULTY
	20 MINUTES + 2 TO 3 WEEKS	2 QUARTS	●●○○

4 to 5 pounds cabbage (about 2 medium heads)

2 tablespoons sea salt

You also need:

2 1-quart glass jars with airlocks

Clean fermenting weights or stones

Tamper (optional)

1 Finely shred the cabbage and place it in a bowl in batches, sprinkling each batch with a layer of sea salt. When you are finished with the shredding, use your hands to massage the cabbage well until it breaks down and becomes soft (about 10 minutes). Let the massaged cabbage sit for 10 minutes to let it release its juices.

2 Pack the cabbage very tightly into jars, pushing all of it down until it is completely submerged by its own juices (a tamper is helpful here). Leave about an inch and a half head space, and add some additional brine (made by dissolving 1 teaspoon sea salt in 1 cup of water) if there is not enough liquid to fully submerge the cabbage. Place the fermenting stones on top to weigh down the cabbage, tighten the lid and ensure the airlock is installed properly (refer to the instructions that came with your unit, as they can vary). It is possible to ferment without an airlock; be sure to check out some of the online resources on page 304 for further information.

3 Let the cabbage ferment at room temperature for 2 to 3 weeks; during this time, the sauerkraut will bubble a little and intensify in flavor. If any scum appears, remove it with a spoon. Taste it starting at two weeks, and when the taste is to your liking, you can remove the airlock, put a regular lid on the jars and store in the refrigerator.

Variations: The possibilities for varying your fermented vegetables are endless—you can use different types of cabbage, carrots, beets, garlic, ginger, and many other vegetables in different combinations to make a rich array of tasty probiotic foods. Check the resources on page 304 for links to great websites dedicated to fermentation.

Storage: The sauerkraut will keep for a few months in the refrigerator.

KOMBUCHA

TOOLS	TIME	YIELD	DIFFICULTY
	1 TO 3 WEEKS	1 GALLON	◑○○○

1 gallon filtered water

5 bags of green tea

1 cup granulated sugar
(don't use honey or agave here)

1 kombucha starter culture*

1 cup starter liquid (this should
either come with the starter
culture or be from a previous
batch – if you don't have either
you can use apple cider vinegar)

You will also need:

A 1-gallon glass container
Cheesecloth
Large rubber band

For bottle-fermenting:

Glass jars with lids
Fruit juice

1 Bring the gallon of water to a boil, turn off the heat and add the tea bags. Steep for a minute or two and remove.

2 Add the sugar and stir to combine. Let cool completely to room temperature.

3 When the sweetened tea has cooled, pour it into your gallon container with the starter culture and starter liquid (don't do this before it is cooled—you will kill your culture!). Cover with a cheesecloth secured with a rubber band and let the jar sit in a dark corner at room temperature (about 65 to 75 degrees).

4 You can choose to let your culture ferment for at least a week up to a few weeks, with it getting less sweet and more sour toward the end, as the bacteria eats up most of the sugar. Taste it, and when you like the result, pour most of the kombucha, sparing the culture, into jars and store them in the refrigerator. Leave a couple of cups of liquid in the bottom of the jar to start the next batch. You will also want to remove the new culture that has formed on the top and use to start another batch, or you could give it to a friend!

Bottle Fermenting: To make your kombucha fizzy, put an ounce or two of fresh fruit juice in the bottom of a few quart-size glass jars and fill them to within an inch of the top of the jars with kombucha. You can use any type of juice you like here—pineapple, grape, and pomegranate are some of my favorites. You can also add spices like ginger, turmeric, or clove. Screw the lids on tightly and allow the liquid to ferment at room temperature for a couple of days, being sure to open the lids and "burp" them once a day. When they are finished, put in the refrigerator end enjoy.

*Note: You can find a starter culture (called a scoby) at some natural groceries as well as online, but the best source is to find someone you know locally who can give you a "baby" from a successful culture. The scoby looks like an opaque, jello-like glob and should come accompanied by some starter liquid. Once you make your kombucha for the first time, you will end up with an extra scoby to start a double batch or give to a friend!

Storage: Kombucha keeps for a few months in the refrigerator.

WATER KEFIR

TOOLS	TIME	YIELD	DIFFICULTY
	1 TO 2 DAYS	2 QUARTS	●○○○

2 quarts filtered water, at room temperature

½ cup granulated sugar (do not use honey or agave here)

¼ cup water-kefir grains*

You will also need:

2 quart-size glass jars
Cheesecloth
Rubber bands

1 Place ¼ cup of the sugar in each of the glass jars and add a little bit of warm water to dissolve.

2 Divide the rest of the water between the jars, making sure it is at room temperature (if it is too warm it will kill the grains).

3 Add the grains, cover each jar with a cheesecloth and secure with a rubber band.

4 Place on the counter for 24 to 48 hours to ferment—you should see some bubbles and it will smell slightly sour.

5 Strain out the kefir grains, bottle the liquid, and store in the refrigerator to stop the fermentation. Your kefir is ready to drink as-is or bottle ferment, and you can now use the grains to start another batch.

Bottle Fermenting: To make the kefir carbonated, put the strained water kefir back in the jars with an ounce or two of fruit juice in the bottom. Place an air-tight lid on and let bottle-ferment for a couple of days on the countertop, remembering to "burp" or open the lids once a day to let gases escape. When they are finished, put into the refrigerator and enjoy!

*Note: You can find starter cultures (also called "grains") at some natural groceries and online—or you may have a friend who has a batch that has multiplied. The grains resemble a jelly cottage cheese and may increase in numbers with subsequent batches. If you buy online, sometimes the cultures come dehydrated, so you will need to follow the rehydrating instructions before following this recipe.

Storage: Water kefir keeps for a month in the refrigerator.

RENDERED ANIMAL FAT

TOOLS	TIME	YIELD	DIFFICULTY
	2 TO 4 HOURS	2 CUPS	●●○○

1 pound animal fat (lard, tallow, duck fat, or suet work well), cold

¼ cup water

1 Cut the fat into small pieces—ideally smaller than 1 inch. Place them in a large cast-iron pot or a crockpot with the water and turn the heat to the lowest setting.

2 Let the fat cook on low for an hour or so, stirring every so often.

3 Once there is a considerable amount of fat melted (maybe a third to a half of the solid fat), strain most of it through a fine mesh strainer into another pot, leaving about 1/4 cup in with the solid fat and set aside. Place the remaining un-rendered fat back on the stove. Continue doing this until there is only a small amount of un-rendered fat in the pot.

4 Once all of the fat is in the second pot and warm enough to be liquefied but not still hot, transfer into a glass jar for storage.

Note: You can take the solids (the cracklings) left in the pot after the rendering process and bake them for 20 minutes at 400 degrees. They make a great crunchy snack or salad topping!

Sourcing Note: Make sure to use fat from healthy animals—those that have been raised on pasture and fed an appropriate diet.

Storage: Keeps for a few months in the refrigerator. Also freezes well.

COCONUT CONCENTRATE

TOOLS	TIME	YIELD	DIFFICULTY
	10 MINUTES	1½ CUPS	●●○○

4 cups dried, fine shredded coconut (unsweetened)
1 tablespoon coconut oil
Sea salt to taste

You will also need:

High-powered blender or food processor

1 Place the coconut flakes, coconut oil, and salt in the blender.

2 Process on high speed, while pushing down with a tamper (you may have to stop and do this manually if you are using a food processor). Process for about a minute at a time, taking breaks so as to not overheat the motor. After about 5 to 10 minutes, you should be left with a thick, creamy paste.

3 Pour into a glass jar.

Storage: Keeps well at room temperature for a few months.

CREAMY COCONUT MILK

TOOLS	TIME	YIELD	DIFFICULTY
	20 MINUTES	1½ CUPS	●●○○

1 cup fine shredded coconut
   (unsweetened)
2 cups boiling filtered water
Sea salt to taste

You will also need:

Blender
Cheesecloth

1 Place the shredded coconut and boiling water in your blender and blend on high speed for a few minutes, taking breaks for the motor if needed.

2 Let cool for at least 15 minutes—until it can be safely handled. Strain through a cheesecloth into a glass jar.

Note: Keeps for a few days stored in the refrigerator. The cream will separate from the liquid, so shake or heat gently before using.

RECOMMENDED TOOLS

· Heavy-bottomed pot (Dutch oven) - Having a versatile, heavy-bottomed pot that can go from the stovetop to the oven and has a tight-fitting lid is very handy. Le Creuset and Staub make very nice products, but there are much less expensive alternatives, like Lodge.

· Roasting dish and baking sheets - You will need at least one sturdy baking/cookie sheet and one deep roasting dish.

· Cast-iron skillet – It's great to have a seasoned cast-iron skillet on hand for browning meats and sautéing on the stovetop. Another plus is that it can go in the oven and double as a small roasting dish.

· Chef's knife – You need at least one good, sharp knife for slicing meat and chopping vegetables. For all of the cooking you are going to be doing on the Autoimmune Protocol, it is worth it to have a nice, sharp knife!

· Mixing bowls – You want at least two sizeable mixing bowls (stainless steel is lightweight and durable) for prepping food and tossing salads.

· Spoons and utensils – It's good to have a variety of utensils for cooking. Make sure you have a pair of tongs, a couple of large wooden stirring spoons, a spatula, and a whisk.

· Cutting board – If you are sharing a house with others who may be eating food not included on the protocol, you may want to invest in a separate cutting board. I like wooden boards that have feet so they don't warp with constant washing.

· High-powered blender – This appliance is kind of a splurge, but really makes food prep a lot easier. In addition to making smoothies and sauces like a regular blender, the high-powered variety can handle things like coconut butter, emulsions, sorbet, and thick sauces. I prefer VitaMix, but there are other quality brands out there.

· Glass storage containers - Portion-size glass storage containers are incredibly useful for storing leftovers in the refrigerator. Be sure to get ones with BPA-free lids.

· Meat thermometer – It's a really good idea to have a good meat thermometer, especially if you plan on cooking a lot of poultry.

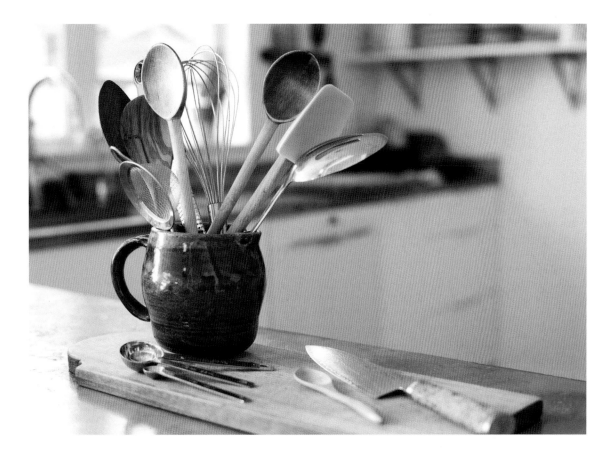

· Little tools – Having some assorted little tools makes some tasks easier—I like having a spiralizer, mandoline, microplane zester, and vegetable peeler. You should also have a set of measuring cups and spoons.

· Extras - Some unnecessary, slightly fancy tools would be a pressure cooker to make bone broth more quickly, a food processor (especially if you don't have a high-powered blender), and a juicer. You definitely don't need these tools to try the Autoimmune Protocol, but they do make some tasks easier.

TIPS + TRICKS

HOW TO USE THIS BOOK

All the recipes in this book are suitable for the Autoimmune Protocol (known in Sarah Ballantyne's work as "The Paleo Approach"). Although most people end up expanding the list of foods they can tolerate, I wanted to create a resource for those at the beginning of the process. If you don't want to jump in right away and instead are interested in a slower transition, I encourage you to try some recipes to get your feet wet—I think you'll be surprised at how easy and palatable they are!

It is my hope that you use the meal plans as a template, making modifications and substitutions as you go to reflect your preferences and the availability of ingredients in your area. I know there are many people with digestive issues who would need to eliminate certain vegetables, and in that case, I want you to get comfortable making additions and substitutions. For instance, if you don't tolerate sweet potato, substitute butternut squash. If you are avoiding onions or garlic, leave them out and substitute ginger. If you prefer Swiss chard over kale, go for it! My goal is to give you the tools to cook simple, flavorful meals that can easily be customized to your preferences or the season.

A Note On Sugar

Although it is well known that sugar can cause autoimmune flares, this is not a completely sugar-free cookbook. I have included some fruit for flavoring within the context of a balanced meal—one with adequate protein and fat. I have also included a small dessert section; most of those recipes are fruit-sweetened, but there are a couple with maple syrup or honey. I don't advise including excessive fruit or sugar (even from natural sources like maple syrup or honey) while on the Autoimmune Protocol, but I wanted to include those recipes for a special occasion or a treat if needed. I guess this is a warning to not go crazy in this department—it will hinder your progress!

A Note On Cooking Fat

Instead of specifying which fat to use in the recipes, I call for "solid cooking fat." This can be any fat of your choosing, as long as it is saturated and solid at room temperature: coconut oil, lard, tallow, duck fat, among others. Sometimes I have specified coconut oil when the recipe requires a more neutral flavor, but don't be afraid to substitute if you would like to use something else. I have included a recipe for rendering your own fat on page 42.

A NOTE ON FOOD QUALITY

The Autoimmune Protocol removes gut irritants and common potential allergens, replacing them with whole, nourishing foods and thereby removing all of the commercial processed foods that are so prevalent in our modern society. Simply avoiding certain foods and eating others is not the entire plan, however—food quality plays a critical role when you are on a mission to heal and nourish your body. It is well known that the nutritional value of food can vary greatly, depending on how it was grown or raised—and when our goal is to seek out those nutrients that enable our bodies to heal, the search to find high-quality food becomes very important.

Before you run off to your local natural grocer and pay top dollar for products that are raised organically/pastured/grass-fed, you may want to do some research into what is available locally and seasonally to cut down on costs (and often times these products end up being more healthy for us *and* the planet!). If you're on a budget and can't afford the highest quality of everything, prioritize and go from there. Don't assume that because you can't afford natural-market prices for high quality food it is out of your budget. Buying in bulk, shopping seasonally, volunteering at a farmers' market, shopping online, starting a garden, and frequenting a few different stores are all smart strategies that will cut costs while keeping food quality high.

SHOPPING GUIDE

Meat: It is very important to buy hormone-free meat, at the very least. Of course organic, grass-fed, and pastured are preferable, but it is unrealistic to expect that everyone has the access or budget to afford it. If you can't afford grass-fed or pastured all the time, try buying the tougher, fattier cuts of meat (which are usually cheaper anyway) grass-fed and the leaner cuts at least hormone-free. Also, buying in bulk directly from a farmer saves a ton over paying premium prices at the store—check out the resources on page 304 to find a farm near you. A deep freezer is great for storing a bulk meat order, as well as a place to freeze extra meat you might find on sale at the store or farmers' market. In the case of fish, always be sure to buy wild-caught varieties—not farmed. Canned fish should be packed in BPA-free cans and free of fillers and other ingredients.

Fats/Oils: Olive and avocado oils are the only unsaturated oils (liquid at room temperature) that I recommend on the Autoimmune Protocol. Do not buy any nut or seed oils (sesame, walnut, canola). Be sure to buy brands that are cold-pressed and come in opaque bottles. Only use liquid oils for cold applications, like salad dressings or to drizzle on raw vegetables. For cooking, always use some form of solid fat, either of tropical or animal origin. Coconut oil is a great staple for cooking and one I use often in my kitchen. Animal fats are also a good choice, as long as they come from a good source (pastured animals), as toxins are often stored in the fat. If you are willing to render your own fat (page 42), chunks of lard, tallow, and sometimes duck fat can be purchased from many farmers quite inexpensively.

Produce: If you cannot get all organic produce, use the reference lists of the most toxic non-organic produce to guide your purchases. Buying locally and in season is always preferable and usually the most cost-effective. If you have a cool place to store them, root vegetables like squashes, sweet potatoes, and onions can be purchased in bulk. Farmer's markets and CSAs are always the best source for produce if you can manage to find one in your area, followed by natural grocers. Don't assume that you have to travel great distances to find organic produce these days, as most conventional supermarkets have increasingly more varieties and better prices on organic goods.

A NOTE ON BATCH COOKING

One of the biggest ways to make the Autoimmune Protocol go more smoothly is to incorporate weekly batch cooking into your routine, especially if you are crunched for time during the work week. Because the Autoimmune Protocol excludes all processed foods, everything must be cooked from scratch. This can be extremely problematic for someone who works full time, cares for children, or is very ill. On the next page, I have compiled some ideas to get you started on planning a batch-cooking routine and help you make sure that you always have nutrient-dense meal components ready to go.

BATCH-COOKING IDEAS

• **Bone Broth** - Make this once a week (page 34) and store in glass jars for use in soups, stews, and for drinking with breakfast instead of coffee. If you really want to get ahead, make two batches at the same time and freeze one of them.

• **Meat Patties** - Homemade meat patties are the best security blanket on the Autoimmune Protocol. Make a batch or two once a week and freeze the patties between slices of waxed paper. You can make a few different kinds: Three-Herb Beef (page 262), Garlic-Sage Chicken (page 211), or Rosemary-Mint Lamb (page 269)—then you always have a quick, clean source of protein and some variety to choose from. Homemade meat patties are the fastest protein for breakfast—just reheat them gently in a skillet. You can also use them for a quick meal or a snack if you run short of other options.

• **Soups/Stews** - When making a soup or stew, it's a great idea to double the recipe and freeze half of it in portion-size containers. Then you can pull one out to thaw overnight for a lunch at work or a quick meal.

• **Meat** – It's great to get in the habit of cooking a big batch of meat to add to meals over the following days. For instance, you can make the Herbed Roast Chicken (page 227), pull off all of the meat, and then use the carcass to make bone broth. Then you can reserve the meat to add to salads, lettuce boats, and stir-fries. Making a big batch of Shredded Roast Beef (page 261) or Shredded Chicken Breast (page 212) is also great for this. Save recipes that are time consuming for your batch-cooking day, and then the days following you can just use the meat to assemble meals with some quickly cooked vegetables.

• **Staples** - Make staples like Creamy Coconut Milk (page 46), Coconut Concentrate (page 45), Garlic "Mayo" (page 127), Coconut-Basil Pesto (page 124), Nomato Sauce (page 135) and other dressings and sauces that keep well on your batch-cooking day. Then you'll have an assortment of components to draw on for recipes and meals.

THOUGHTS ON BREAKFAST

When people think of a breakfast, even a so-called "healthy" one, it's hard not to conjure up images containing grains and eggs. The Autoimmune Protocol does not lend itself well to traditional breakfast-type foods, with the possible exceptions of bacon and sausage (and even sausages usually contain nightshade spices). Because of this, I have not included a breakfast category in the cookbook. This is perhaps one of the most difficult concepts for people to get once they decide to start eating this way. The only thing that makes breakfast different from lunch or dinner on this plan is that it is generally a meal that needs to be prepared more quickly than usual. For this reason, it's even more ideal to have pre-prepared meals or components on hand.

I think it is important to make breakfast the most hearty, satisfying meal of the day. I know this is hard for those who are not hungry in the morning, or those who are used to drinking a cup of coffee and running out the door. If you don't like eating breakfast, start increasing the quality and quantity of your morning meal gradually, and you might find that your morning hunger improves. Be sure to include a few ounces of protein and some fat at breakfast, as this is very important to keep your blood sugar stable and keep you satiated for the rest of the day. Remember: Healing bodies need lots of quality fuel, and breakfast is a perfect time to get these nutrients in.

My favorite breakfasts are those that combine foods I have prepared ahead of time, like sausage patties or other protein, leftover vegetables or fresh cooked greens, some fermented vegetables, a mug of bone broth, and maybe a slice of fruit or bacon to round out the plate. All of these items are readily available in my kitchen, and I can easily piece together a nourishing and nutrient-dense meal in a matter of minutes. On the next page I've given you some examples of foods to have available to create a satisfying and healing breakfast.

BREAKFAST IDEAS

- **Meat Patties** - If you have at least two different kinds in your freezer, you can avoid having the same thing for breakfast every morning. Just grab one out of the freezer and reheat it in a skillet. Try the Three-Herb Breakfast Patties (page 262), Garlic-Sage Chicken Patties (page 211), or Rosemary-Mint Lamb Patties (page 269).

- **Bone Broth** - Breakfast is a great time to enjoy a mug of broth! It can replace your morning coffee or tea, or you can add some leftover vegetables and meat to create a quick soup. My recipe is on page 34.

- **Fermented Vegetables** - Sauerkraut (page 37) or other fermented vegetables can be stored in your fridge and just scooped out onto your plate to add to breakfast.

- **Leftover Vegetables** - If you have any leftover veggies from your dinner the day before, you can throw them into the skillet to heat up with the meat patties. You can also batch-cook a big vegetable hash every week to quickly reheat for breakfasts.

- **Raw Fruit or Vegetables** - You can eat a piece of fruit or some raw vegetables with your breakfast, but I would not choose this in lieu of quality protein or fat.

- **Canned Fish** - If you run out of patties or are in a rush, a BPA-free can of fish (salmon or sardines are nice) mashed up with some raw veggies can be a quick solution.

- **Bacon** - Always a nice addition to breakfast. Be sure to purchase the pastured, sugar-free variety.

- **Leftover Meals** - Forget your prior conception of breakfast. If you have a leftover portion of stew or other hearty meal with a serving of protein, eat it for breakfast!

MEAL PLANS

ABOUT THE MEAL PLANS

On the following pages I have included two meal plans that each cover a month's worth of meals, including shopping lists for the corresponding recipes. For these meal plans I've selected recipes that are easy to make, palatable to a wide variety of preferences, and keep well enough to be eaten as leftovers throughout the week. My goal in organizing information this way is to give those who may be new to this style of eating a concrete plan so that they can set themselves up to be successful in their transition. By the end of the month, you should be very comfortable working with a wide range of ingredients and ready to branch out and make your own weekly meal plans. Because most people are busy or work a traditional schedule, I have scheduled the bulk of the cooking to happen on the weekends and at dinnertime. All lunches on the plan are leftovers that may be taken to work or prepared quickly on the go.

The Complete Four-Week Meal Plan is what I would recommend for those coming to the Autoimmune Protocol for the first time, especially if they are transitioning from a standard American diet. This is a very plentiful, nourishing diet, and I have erred on the side of caution when planning food portions—there should be more food rather than not enough. Changing to a very restrictive diet can be challenging if there is not enough food available, and I have allowed so that a person following this plan will always have some extra food available in case they get hungry between meals.

The Alternate Four-Week Meal Plan is for those who don't want to eat meat at every meal, for either personal preference or because of budget concerns. Although I recommend having at least a small serving of meat at every meal, I wanted to make a plan for those who could only afford a certain amount of high-quality meat or were put off by the thought of eating so much of it. This plan is similar to the complete plan except that there is no meat at lunchtime.

A FEW NOTES BEFORE YOU START

• The meal plans account for one person for four weeks. As I said previously, the plans both account for generous servings of food, in an effort to avoid a situation where a person is hungry but doesn't have anything available to eat. If you find that you have excess food prepared, drop some of the vegetable side dishes and eat leftovers instead.

• Meals that need to be cooked from scratch are denoted in color and correspond to page numbers for the recipes in the book. You can easily glance at the week and see which meals you will need to cook from scratch. All of the meals in black have already been prepped or cooked previously and should only take a quick re-heat or assembly.

• I have accounted for 4 to 6 ounces of meat per meal in the shopping lists. If you want to be eating more or less, adjust your shopping list and recipes accordingly.

• There are twice-weekly shopping lists that take into consideration how long the meat will last in the refrigerator, but you have the option of buying all the meat for a week and then freezing some portions for later. Generally meat takes 24 to 48 hours to thaw in the refrigerator, so plan accordingly; you want to have your meat ready to go when you're ready to cook.

• There is a list of pantry items to be stocked while on the meal plan on each shopping list. These are items that store well and are commonly used—like onions, vinegar and sea salt. It is assumed that as you run out of them, you will stock up.

• For breakfasts, I have only included the meat component. I suggest completing the meal with leftover vegetables, fermented vegetables, bone broth, or items like avocados, bacon, or fruit. Getting in the hang of assembling a great breakfast takes some planning, but after a few days you will find a combination and amount that suits you and fuels your day.

COMPLETE 4-WEEK MEAL PLAN

WEEK 1

	BREAKFAST	LUNCH	DINNER
SUNDAY	Three-Herb Beef Patties (page 262) (also make Garlic-Sage Chicken Patties page 211)	Citrus-Ginger Marinated Salmon (page 237) Cauliflower "Fried Rice" (page 200)	Classic Chicken Soup (page 165)*
MONDAY	Three-Herb Beef Patties	Classic Chicken Soup	Citrus-Ginger Marinated Salmon Cauliflower "Fried Rice"
TUESDAY	Garlic-Sage Chicken Patties	Citrus-Ginger Marinated Salmon Cauliflower "Fried Rice"	Garlic Beef and Broccoli (page 270)*** Radish and Jicama Tabbouli (page 142)
WEDNESDAY	Mediterranean Salmon Salad (page 153)	Classic Chicken Soup	Shredded Chicken Breast (page 212) Curried Chicken Salad (page 224) Emerald Kale Salad (page 138)
THURSDAY	Mediterranean Salmon Salad	Garlic Beef and Broccoli Radish and Jicama Tabbouli	Curried Chicken Salad Emerald Kale Salad
FRIDAY	Three-Herb Beef Patties	Curried Chicken Salad Emerald Kale Salad	Mediterranean Salmon (page 242) Rosemary Grilled Asparagus (page 195) Sautéed Market Greens (page 183)
SATURDAY	Three-Herb Beef Patties	Mediterranean Salmon Rosemary Grilled Asparagus Sautéed Market Greens	Beef-Butternut Stew with Pear and Thyme (page 161)**

*Freeze two servings **Freeze one serving ***Halve recipe

WEEK 2

	BREAKFAST	LUNCH	DINNER
SUNDAY	Garlic-Sage Chicken Patties	Mediterranean Salmon Rosemary Grilled Asparagus Sautéed Market Greens	Beef-Butternut Stew with Pear and Thyme Shredded Roast Beef (page 261) (save for later in week)**
MONDAY	Mediterranean Salmon Salad (page 153)	Beef-Butternut Stew with Pear and Thyme	Shredded Chicken Breast (page 212) Chicken Stir-Fry (page 231) Curried Cauliflower (page 187)
TUESDAY	Mediterranean Salmon Salad	Chicken Stir-Fry Curried Cauliflower	Coconut Amino–Marinated Salmon (page 237) Cabbage Slaw with Olive-Avocado Dressing (page 145)
WEDNESDAY	Garlic-Sage Chicken Patties	Coconut Amino–Marinated Salmon Cabbage Slaw with Olive-Avocado Dressing	Rosemary Shredded Beef Skillet (page 278) Emerald Kale Salad (page 138)
THURSDAY	Garlic-Sage Chicken Patties	Coconut Amino–Marinated Salmon Cabbage Slaw with Olive-Avocado Dressing	Rosemary Shredded Beef Skillet Emerald Kale Salad
FRIDAY	Garlic-Sage Chicken Patties	Rosemary Shredded Beef Skillet Emerald Kale Salad	Asian Marinated Grilled Chicken (page 219) Carrot-Ginger Soup (page 162)*
SATURDAY	Three-Herb Beef Patties (page 262) (also make Garlic-Sage Chicken Patties page 211)	Asian Marinated Grilled Chicken Carrot-Ginger Soup	Citrus-Ginger Marinated Salmon (page 237) Market Salad (page 149)

*Freeze one serving **Halve recipe

COMPLETE 4-WEEK MEAL PLAN

WEEK 3

	BREAKFAST	LUNCH	DINNER
SUNDAY	Garlic-Sage Chicken Patties	Citrus-Ginger Marinated Salmon Market Salad	Cinnamon-Sage Dry-Rub Steak (page 265)** Brussels Sprouts with Crispy Bacon (page 191)
MONDAY	Three-Herb Beef Patties	Cinnamon-Sage Dry-Rub Steak Brussels Sprouts with Crispy Bacon	Lemon-Garlic Marinated Chicken (page 219) Market Salad
TUESDAY	Three-Herb Beef Patties	Lemon-Garlic Marinated Chicken Brussels Sprouts with Crispy Bacon	Classic Tuna Salad (page 232) Mashed Sweet Potatoes (page 192)*
WEDNESDAY	Mediterranean Salmon Salad (page 153)	Classic Tuna Salad Mashed Sweet Potatoes	Classic Chicken Soup (frozen; thawed day prior)
THURSDAY	Mediterranean Salmon Salad	Classic Chicken Soup (frozen; thawed two days prior)	Shredded Chicken Breast (page 212) Chicken and Pesto Sauté (page 216) Rainbow Roasted Root Vegetables (page 188)
FRIDAY	Three-Herb Beef Patties	Classic Tuna Salad Mashed Sweet Potatoes	Chicken and Pesto Sauté Rainbow Roasted Root Vegetables
SATURDAY	Garlic-Sage Chicken Patties	Sole Fillet with Tarragon-Caper Sauce (page 245) Puréed Parsnips (page 196)	Herbed Dry-Rub Steak (page 265)** Sautéed Market Greens (page 183) Rainbow Roasted Root Vegetables

*Thaw two servings of soup **Halve recipe

WEEK 4

	BREAKFAST	LUNCH	DINNER
SUNDAY	Garlic-Sage Chicken Patties	Sole Fillet with Tarragon-Caper Sauce Sautéed Market Greens Puréed Parsnips	Shredded Roast Beef (page 261) Lettuce Boats Mango Salsa (page 131)
MONDAY	Garlic-Sage Chicken Patties	Shredded Roast Beef Lettuce Boats Mango Salsa	Sole Fillet with Tarragon-Caper Sauce Sautéed Market Greens Puréed Parsnips
TUESDAY	Mediterranean Salmon Salad (page 153)	Shredded Roast Beef Lettuce Boats Mango Salsa	Sage-Braised Chicken Legs (page 228)** Puréed Parsnips (page 196)
WEDNESDAY	Mediterranean Salmon Salad	Sage-Braised Chicken Legs Puréed Parsnips	"Spaghetti" and Meatballs (page 282)** Cinnamon-Scented Butternut Squash (page 184)
THURSDAY	Three-Herb Beef Patties	"Spaghetti" and Meatballs Cinnamon-Scented Butternut Squash	Salmon Salad with Olives and Cucumber (page 238) Cucumber-Mint Salad (page 141)*
FRIDAY	Garlic-Sage Chicken Patties	Salmon Salad with Olives and Cucumber Cucumber-Mint Salad	Beef-Butternut Stew with Pear and Thyme (frozen; thawed day prior) Cinnamon-Scented Butternut Squash*
SATURDAY	Garlic-Sage Chicken Patties	Salmon Salad with Olives and Cucumber Emerald Kale Salad (page 138)	Herbed Dry-Rub Steak (page 265)*** Carrot-Ginger Soup (frozen; thawed day prior) Emerald Kale Salad

*Thaw one serving of soup **Halve recipe ***Quarter recipe

COMPLETE 4-WEEK MEAL PLAN

PANTRY ITEMS	WEEK 1	WEEK 2
	SATURDAY	**SATURDAY**
solid cooking fat of your choice (lard, tallow, duck fat, etc) coconut oil extra-virgin olive oil coconut cream ginger powder turmeric powder sage powder cinnamon powder bay leaves sea salt coconut flour kalamata olives capers apple cider vinegar coconut aminos shredded coconut flakes	2 pounds grass-fed ground beef 2 pounds chicken thigh, ground 1 4-5 pound pastured stewing hen 24 ounces wild salmon 1 pound grass-fed sirloin steak 2 pounds carrots 1 bunch celery 1 bunch radishes 1/2 pound jicama 1 zucchini 2 cucumbers 1 bunch broccoli 1 head cauliflower 1 cup mushrooms 2 pounds green beans 2 oranges fresh chives fresh mint fresh parsley (large bunch) fresh rosemary fresh sage (2 bunches) fresh thyme	2 pound beef roast or stew meat 2 pound beef roast 1 pound wild-caught salmon 1 pound pastured chicken breast 1 large butternut squash 2 pounds carrots 1 lb broccoli 3 cups mushrooms 1 head cauliflower 1 small head savoy cabbage 1-2 avocados 2 firm pears fresh parsley fresh thyme
KEEP IN STOCK	**WEDNESDAY**	**WEDNESDAY**
yellow onions red onions fresh garlic fresh ginger lemons BPA-free canned salmon BPA-free canned tuna	1 pound wild-caught salmon 1 pound pastured chicken breast 1 small cucumber 3 bunches dark leafy greens (kale, chard, collards) 2 pounds asparagus 1 head lettuce fresh parsley fresh rosemary ¼ cup raisins	1 pound pastured chicken breast 2 large sweet potatoes 2 pounds carrots 2 zucchini squash 1 bunch kale 1 small cucumber 1 orange fresh chives fresh rosemary
HAVE READY fermented vegetables (page 37) bone broth (page 34) garlic "mayo" (page 127)		

SHOPPING LIST

WEEK 3	WEEK 4
SATURDAY	**SATURDAY**
2 pounds grass-fed ground beef	2 pound beef roast
2 pounds chicken thigh, ground	12 ounces grass-fed steak
1 pound wild-caught salmon	1 ½ pounds pastured chicken legs
1 pound pastured chicken breast	and thighs
1 pound grass-fed steak	2 large bunches of dark leafy greens
6 slices sugar-free bacon	(kale, collards, chard)
2 pounds sweet potatoes	1 ½ pounds parsnips
1 ½ pounds brussels sprouts	1 head romaine lettuce
½ cup mushrooms	1-2 bunches spinach
1 head lettuce	2 cucumbers
1 head romaine	2 cups mushrooms
3 carrots	1 bunch radishes
1 bunch celery	1 avocado
1 beet	1 mango
1 cucumber	1 lime
1 avocado	fresh cilantro (large bunch)
2 oranges	fresh parsley
fresh dill	fresh sage (2 bunches)
fresh mint	
fresh parsley	
fresh rosemary	
fresh sage	
fresh thyme	
WEDNESDAY	**WEDNESDAY**
1 pound pastured chicken breast	1 pound ground beef
1 pound sole fillets	6 ounces grass-fed steak
1 ½ pounds parsnips	3 pounds butternut squash
1 pound broccoli or broccolini	2 beets
5 carrots	2 carrots
3 beets	4 zucchini
3 parsnips	1 bunch curly-leafed kale
1 rutabaga	1 bunch mixed greens or lettuce
fresh basil (2 bunches)	1 cucumber
fresh tarragon	fresh basil (large bunch)
½ cup coconut water (optional)	fresh parsley
	fresh rosemary
	fresh sage
	fresh thyme

ALTERNATE 4-WEEK MEAL PLAN

WEEK 1

	BREAKFAST	LUNCH	DINNER
SUNDAY	Three-Herb Beef Patties (page 262) (also make Garlic-Sage Chicken Patties page 211)	Hearty Vegetable Soup (page 173)*	Citrus-Ginger Marinated Salmon (page 237) Rosemary-Roasted Carrots and Parsnips (page 203) Sautéed Market Greens (page 183)
MONDAY	Three-Herb Beef Patties	Hearty Vegetable Soup	Citrus-Ginger Marinated Salmon Rosemary-Roasted Carrots and Parsnips
TUESDAY	Garlic-Sage Chicken Patties	Hearty Vegetable Soup	Garlic Beef and Broccoli (page 270)*** Cauliflower "Fried Rice" (page 200)
WEDNESDAY	Mediterranean Salmon Salad (page 153)	Cauliflower "Fried Rice" Sautéed Market Greens	Garlic Beef and Broccoli Mashed Sweet Potatoes (page 192)
THURSDAY	Mediterranean Salmon Salad	Cauliflower "Fried Rice" Mashed Sweet Potatoes	Shredded Chicken Breast (page 212) Curried Chicken Salad (page 224) Emerald Kale Salad (page 138)
FRIDAY	Three-Herb Beef Patties	Emerald Kale Salad Mashed Sweet Potatoes	Curried Chicken Salad Radish and Jicama Tabbouli (page 142)
SATURDAY	Garlic-Sage Chicken Patties	Emerald Kale Salad Radish and Jicama Tabbouli	Beef-Butternut Stew with Pear and Thyme (page 161)**

*Freeze three servings of soup **Freeze two servings of soup ***Halve recipe

WEEK 2

	BREAKFAST	LUNCH	DINNER
SUNDAY	Garlic-Sage Chicken Patties	Rainbow Roasted Root Vegetables (page 188) Radish and Jicama Tabbouli	Beef-Butternut Stew with Pear and Thyme Cabbage Slaw with Olive-Avocado Dressing (page 145) (prep for lunches later in week)
MONDAY	Mediterranean Salmon Salad (page 153)	Cabbage Slaw with Olive-Avocado Dressing Rainbow Roasted Root Vegetables	Beef-Butternut Stew with Pear and Thyme
TUESDAY	Mediterranean Salmon Salad	Cabbage Slaw with Olive-Avocado Dressing Rainbow Roasted Root Vegetables	"Spaghetti" and Meatballs (page 282)* Carrot-Ginger Soup (page 162)
WEDNESDAY	Garlic-Sage Chicken Patties	Cabbage Slaw with Olive-Avocado Dressing Carrot-Ginger Soup	"Spaghetti" and Meatballs Rosemary Grilled Asparagus (page 195)
THURSDAY	Three-Herb Beef Patties	Carrot-Ginger Soup Rosemary Grilled Asparagus	Mediterranean Salmon (page 242) Citrus-Spinach Salad (page 150) Sautéed Market Greens (page 183)
FRIDAY	Garlic-Sage Chicken Patties	Citrus-Spinach Salad Rosemary Grilled Asparagus	Mediterranean Salmon Sautéed Market Greens Puréed Parsnips (page 196)
SATURDAY	Three-Herb Beef Patties (page 262) (also make Garlic-Sage Chicken Patties page 211)	Citrus-Spinach Salad Sautéed Market Greens	Mediterranean Salmon Puréed Parsnips Cinnamon-Scented Butternut Squash (page 184)

*Halve recipe

ALTERNATE 4-WEEK MEAL PLAN

WEEK 3

	BREAKFAST	LUNCH	DINNER
SUNDAY	Garlic-Sage Chicken Patties	Cinnamon-Scented Butternut Squash Puréed Parsnips	Lemon-Garlic Marinated Chicken (page 219) Emerald Kale Salad (page 138)
MONDAY	Three-Herb Beef Patties	Cinnamon-Scented Butternut Squash Emerald Kale Salad	Lemon-Garlic Marinated Chicken Beet and Fennel Soup (page 162)*
TUESDAY	Three-Herb Beef Patties	Cinnamon-Scented Butternut Squash Emerald Kale Salad	Classic Tuna Salad (page 234) Market Salad (page 149)
WEDNESDAY	Mediterranean Salmon Salad (page 153)	Beet and Fennel Soup Market Salad	Classic Tuna Salad Mashed Sweet Potatoes (page 192)
THURSDAY	Mediterranean Salmon Salad	Hearty Vegetable Soup (frozen; thawed the day prior) Market Salad	Classic Tuna Salad Mashed Sweet Potatoes Roasted Mixed Vegetables (page 199)**
FRIDAY	Three-Herb Beef Patties	Mashed Sweet Potatoes Roasted Mixed Vegetables	Beef-Butternut Stew with Pear and Thyme (frozen; thawed the day prior)
SATURDAY	Garlic-Sage Chicken Patties	Curried Cauliflower (page 187) Roasted Mixed Vegetables	Beef-Butternut Stew with Pear and Thyme (frozen; thawed two days prior)

*Freeze one serving of soup **Freeze two servings of soup

WEEK 4

	BREAKFAST	LUNCH	DINNER
SUNDAY	Three-Herb Beef Patties	Curried Cauliflower Market Salad (page 149)	Sole Fillet with Tarragon-Caper Sauce (page 245) Emerald Kale Salad (page 138)* Market Salad
MONDAY	Garlic-Sage Chicken Patties	Emerald Kale Salad Hearty Vegetable Soup (frozen; thawed the day prior)	Sole Fillet with Tarragon-Caper Sauce Cucumber-Mint Salad (page 141)
TUESDAY	Mediterranean Salmon Salad (page 153)	Cucumber-Mint Salad Hearty Vegetable Soup (frozen; thawed two days prior)	Sole Fillet with Tarragon-Caper Sauce Brussels Sprouts with Crispy Bacon (page 191)**
WEDNESDAY	Mediterranean Salmon Salad	Beet and Fennel Soup Brussels Sprouts with Crispy Bacon	Sage-Braised Chicken Legs (page 228)*** Puréed Parsnips (page 196) Sautéed Market Greens (page 183)
THURSDAY	Three-Herb Beef Patties	Puréed Parsnips Sautéed Market Greens	Sage-Braised Chicken Legs Brussels Sprouts with Crispy Bacon Rainbow Roasted Root Vegetables (page 188)
FRIDAY	Garlic-Sage Chicken Patties	Sautéed Market Greens Rainbow Roasted Root Vegetables	Coconut Amino–Marinated Salmon (page 237) Cauliflower "Fried Rice" (page 200) Rosemary Grilled Asparagus (page 195)
SATURDAY	Garlic-Sage Chicken Patties	Rainbow Roasted Root Vegetables Rosemary Grilled Asparagus	Coconut Amino–Marinated Salmon Cauliflower "Fried Rice"

*Thaw two servings of soup **Thaw one serving of soup ***Halve recipe

ALTERNATE 4-WEEK MEAL PLAN

	WEEK 1	WEEK 2
PANTRY ITEMS	**SATURDAY**	**SATURDAY**
solid cooking fat of your choice (lard, tallow, duck fat, etc) coconut oil extra-virgin olive oil coconut cream ginger powder turmeric powder sage powder cinnamon powder bay leaves sea salt coconut flour kalamata olives capers apple cider vinegar coconut aminos shredded coconut flakes	2 pounds grass-fed ground beef 2 pounds pastured chicken thigh, ground 1 pound wild-caught salmon 1 pound grass-fed sirloin steak 1 bunch broccolini or broccoli 1 large head cauliflower 2 bunches dark leafy greens (kale, chard, collard greens) 1 bunch chard 3 pounds carrots 1 ½ pounds parsnips 1 zucchini 1 sweet potato 2 cups mushrooms fresh sage (2 bunches) 2 oranges fresh chives fresh mint fresh rosemary fresh thyme	2 pounds grass-fed beef roast or stew meat 1 pound ground beef 1 head savoy cabbage 1 large butternut squash 3 pounds carrots 2 pounds beets 3 parsnips 1 rutabaga 4 zucchini 1 or 2 avocados 2 firm pears 1 cup mushrooms fresh parsley fresh rosemary fresh sage fresh thyme
KEEP IN STOCK	**WEDNESDAY**	**WEDNESDAY**
yellow onions red onions fresh garlic fresh ginger lemons BPA-free canned salmon BPA-free canned tuna	1 pound pastured chicken breast 1 bunch curly-leafed kale 1 ½ pounds sweet potatoes 1 head lettuce 1 bunch radishes 2 cucumbers ½ pound jicama fresh mint fresh parsley ¼ cup raisins	1 pound wild-caught salmon 2 bunches dark green leafy (kale, collard greens, chard) 1-2 bunches spinach 2 pounds parsnips 2 carrots 2 pounds asparagus 1 cucumber 1 avocado 1 orange fresh parsley fresh rosemary
HAVE READY fermented vegetables (page 37) bone broth (page 34) garlic "mayo" (page 127)		

SHOPPING LIST

WEEK 3	WEEK 4
SATURDAY	**SATURDAY**
2 pounds grass-fed ground beef 2 pounds pastured chicken thigh, ground 1 pound pastured chicken breast 3 pounds butternut squash 3 pounds beets 1 large fennel bulb 2 heads of lettuce 1 bunch kale 4 carrots 2 cucumbers 1 avocado fresh dill fresh parsley fresh rosemary fresh sage (2 bunches) fresh thyme	1 pound sole 6 slices sugar-free bacon 1 bunch curly-leafed kale 1 ½ pounds brussels sprouts 1 head lettuce 2 carrots 1 beet 3 cucumbers ½ cup mushrooms 1 avocado fresh mint fresh parsley fresh tarragon
WEDNESDAY	**WEDNESDAY**
2 pounds sweet potatoes 1 bunch celery 1 head cauliflower 4 zucchini 2 portobello mushroom caps fresh rosemary	1 pound pastured chicken legs and thighs 1 pound wild-caught salmon 2 bunches dark leafy greens (kale, collards, chard) 2 pounds asparagus 1 head cauliflower 3 pounds parsnips 6 carrots 3 beets 1 rutabaga 1 zucchini 3 cups mushrooms 1 orange fresh chives fresh rosemary fresh sage (2 bunches)

RECIPES

APPETIZERS + SNACKS

CRISPY KALE CHIPS

TOOLS | TIME | YIELD | DIFFICULTY

30 MINUTES

2 SERVINGS

1 bunch lacinato kale, chopped
   into 2-inch pieces
2 tablespoons coconut oil,
   melted
Sea salt

1 Preheat the oven to 300 degrees F.

2 Place the kale in a large bowl and coat with the coconut oil, stirring to cover all surfaces.

3 Arrange the kale pieces on two or three baking sheets, making sure to leave plenty of space between the pieces.

4 Bake for 20 minutes or until crispy. Remove from the sheet and add salt to taste. Let cool completely (the chips will crisp more as they cool) and serve.

Note: The trick to crispy kale chips is to make sure the kale is completely dry when it goes into the oven, and to salt it only after baking, as the salt will draw moisture out of the leaves, resulting in soggy chips. I like making these with lacinato kale, but feel free to use any variety you have available.

Storage: Keeps sealed in an airtight container at room temperature for several days.

FIG ENERGY BITES

TOOLS | TIME | YIELD | DIFFICULTY
1 HOUR | **16** BITES | ●●○○

2 cups unsulphured dried figs
2 cups fine shredded coconut,
   divided (unsweetened)
⅓ cup coconut oil, melted
¼ teaspoon cinnamon
Pinch of sea salt

1 Place the figs, 1 ½ cups of the shredded coconut, coconut oil, cinnamon, and salt in a food processor and pulse on and off until a thick paste forms (you may have to stop and scrape the sides of your food processor a couple of times).

2 Form into 1-inch balls, then roll them in the reserved ½ cup of shredded coconut.

3 Refrigerate for at least 30 minutes to let the coconut oil set.

Note: Feel free to play around with the dried fruit in this recipe—dates, dried apples, and apricots are all good substitutions for the figs.

Storage: Keeps for a week or two stored in the refrigerator. Also freezes well.

NECTARINE, ARUGULA, AND PROSCIUTTO WRAPS

TOOLS   TIME   YIELD   DIFFICULTY

4

20 MINUTES   SERVINGS   ●○○○

2 nectarines, pitted and cut
   into eighths
1 cup arugula
4 ounces thin-sliced prosciutto

1 Hold a slice of nectarine in your hand and place a few sprigs of arugula alongside it. Use a partial slice of prosciutto to hold them together by wrapping it around the nectarine, about halfway up. The little tufts of arugula will stick out the top.

2 Arrange on a serving platter.

Variation: Use any other stone fruit in place of the nectarine–peaches, plums, and apricots all work well for this recipe.

OLIVE TAPENADE

TOOLS   TIME   YIELD   DIFFICULTY

5 MINUTES   1½ CUPS

1 cup pitted kalamata olives

2 tablespoons capers

3 tablespoons extra-virgin olive oil

2 cloves garlic

¼ cup fresh parsley, lightly packed

Slices of fresh carrot, cucumber, or Rainbow Root Vegetable Chips (page 95)

1 Place the olives, capers, olive oil, garlic, and parsley in a blender or food processor. Blend on low speed for a few seconds, until a thick paste forms. If it is too thick, add an extra tablespoon of olive oil.

2 Serve with fresh vegetable slices or root vegetable chips.

Variation: For a fancier preparation, serve a spoonful of tapenade on a cucumber slice, topped with a sprig of parsley.

Storage: Keeps in the refrigerator for several days.

BACON–BEEF LIVER PATÉ WITH ROSEMARY AND THYME

TOOLS   TIME   YIELD   DIFFICULTY

30 MINUTES   **2** CUPS   ●●●○

6 slices sugar-free bacon

1 small onion, minced

4 cloves garlic, minced

1 pound grass-fed beef liver, rinsed, dried, and sliced into 2- to 3-inch pieces

2 tablespoons minced fresh rosemary

2 tablespoons minced fresh thyme

⅓ cup coconut oil, melted

½ teaspoon sea salt

Fresh herbs, for garnish

Slices of fresh carrot or cucumber, for garnish

1 Cook the bacon slices in a cast-iron skillet, flipping as needed. Cook until crispy. Transfer to a paper towel–lined plate to cool, reserving the fat in the pan.

2 Add the onion and cook for about 5 minutes, stirring, on medium-high heat. Add the garlic and cook for a minute, then add the liver, rosemary, and thyme. Cook 2 to 5 minutes per side, or until the liver is no longer pink in the center. Set aside to cool for a few minutes.

3 Transfer the mixture into a blender* or food processor with the coconut oil and sea salt. Process until it forms a thick paste.

4 Place the paté into a small bowl. Chop the cooled bacon into fine pieces and combine with the paté.

5 Garnish with the fresh herbs and serve with vegetable slices.

*Note: This recipe is difficult to make in a standard blender—you really need a high-powered machine with a tamper for best results.

Storage: Keeps in the refrigerator for several days. Also freezes well.

RAINBOW ROOT VEGETABLE CHIPS

TOOLS　　TIME　　YIELD　　DIFFICULTY

45 MINUTES

3 CUPS

●●●○

**¾ pound root vegetables,
　thinly sliced***
Solid cooking fat, for frying
Sea salt

1 Attach a deep-fry thermometer to the side of a deep, heavy pot. Add enough solid cooking fat to make about 1 ½ inches of melted fat. Heat over medium heat until the fat reaches 350 degrees F. You want to be careful not to get the oil too hot, as it will burn the chips.

2 Fry the chips in batches by type, as they have different cooking times depending on how much moisture they contain. When you first drop the vegetable slices in the oil they will bubble like crazy; after a minute or two of cooking, they will start to bubble less and puff up in the middle. At this point, give them a flip, and continue cooking until the bubbling dies down a lot. When it is apparent they don't have any moisture left, they are finished cooking.

3 Using a slotted spoon, carefully transfer the chips to a paper towel–lined plate and sprinkle with salt to taste. Bring the oil temperature back up to 350 degrees and continue in this fashion until all the chips are cooked.

***Note:** I recommend using a mandoline to get consistently thin slices for this recipe. Your chips will cook more evenly, and chopping will be a lot less work! I also recommend using a deep-fry thermometer to ensure that the oil temperature stays consistent.

Variations: You can use any type of root vegetables for this recipe: sweet potato, carrots, beets, parsnips, turnips, and rutabaga all work great. Using a variety makes for a colorful batch!

Storage: Keeps sealed in an airtight container at room temperature for several days.

PARSLEY-GARLIC DIP

TOOLS   TIME   YIELD   DIFFICULTY

15 MINUTES   1 CUP   ●○○○

3 cups loosely packed parsley
    leaves

¼ cup chopped red onion

2 cloves garlic

10 kalamata olives, pitted

¼ teaspoon sea salt

½ cup extra-virgin olive oil

1 lemon, juiced
    (about 2 tablespoons)

Slices of fresh carrot or
    cucumber, or Rainbow Root
    Vegetable Chips (page 95)

1 Combine all ingredients in a high-powered blender or food processor. Blend on low speed for a few seconds until a thick paste forms.

2 Serve on raw vegetable slices or root vegetable chips.

Storage: Keeps for several days in a sealed container in the refrigerator.

BACON-WRAPPED PEARS

TOOLS   TIME   YIELD   DIFFICULTY

1 HOUR   4 SERVINGS

6 slices thick, sugar-free bacon, cut in half lengthwise
2 ripe pears, cored and sliced into six pieces each
Toothpicks
Powdered cinnamon

1 Preheat the oven to 350 degrees F.

2 Wrap each pear slice in bacon, making a figure eight and securing the loose ends of bacon with a toothpick. Dust lightly with cinnamon and place on a rimmed baking sheet.

3 Bake for 35 to 40 minutes, or until the bacon browns and the pears are cooked throughout.

4 Let cool for 10 minutes and serve warm.

Variation: Substitute apples for the pears or switch the flavor profile by using ginger powder instead of cinnamon. If you use apples, be advised they may need longer to cook.

BEVERAGES

COCONUT MILK CHAI

TOOLS	TIME	YIELD	DIFFICULTY
	30 MINUTES	1½ CUPS	●●○○

1 cup fine shredded coconut
   flakes (unsweetened)
1 whole vanilla bean (optional)
¾ teaspoon cinnamon
1 ½-inch piece ginger, peeled
4 dates, pitted
2 cups boiling water
Cheesecloth

1 Place all ingredients in a high-powered blender and blend on high for a minute or two, until thoroughly combined.

2 Let cool for 15 to 20 minutes.

3 When the liquid is cool enough to handle, strain it through a cheesecloth or nut milk bag; squeeze the contents to yield the maximum amount of liquid.

4 Enjoy iced or reheat in a saucepan.

Storage: Keeps in the refrigerator for several days, but the fat may separate – heat gently and whisk to recombine.

BANANA-BLUEBERRY GREEN SMOOTHIE

TOOLS	TIME	YIELD	DIFFICULTY
	5 MINUTES	2 CUPS	●○○○

1 medium banana
1 cup fresh spinach leaves
½ cup blueberries, frozen
2 tablespoons Coconut
   Concentrate (page 45)
¾ cup filtered water
Ice cubes (optional)

1 Place all ingredients in a blender and blend until well incorporated.

2 If you prefer a thicker or colder drink, add a few ice cubes and blend again. Serve immediately.

Variation: You can substitute kale, chard, or other leafy greens for the spinach, or other types of berries for the blueberries. Don't skip the banana or Coconut Concentrate! They make the drink thick and deliciously creamy.

RASPBERRY CREAM SMOOTHIE

TOOLS	TIME	YIELD	DIFFICULTY
	5 MINUTES	2 CUPS	●○○○

1 banana
¾ cup frozen raspberries
2 tablespoons Coconut
   Concentrate (page 45)
¾ cup filtered water
Ice cubes (optional)

1 Place all ingredients in a blender and blend until well incorporated.

2 If you prefer a thicker or colder drink, add a few ice cubes and blend again. Serve immediately.

Variation: Use blueberries, strawberries, or blackberries instead of raspberries.

MANGO DREAM SMOOTHIE

TOOLS	TIME	YIELD	DIFFICULTY
	5 MINUTES	2 CUPS	●○○○

1 cup frozen mango pieces
1 banana
¾ cup filtered water
2 tablespoons coconut oil
1 tablespoon chopped fresh mint
   leaves (optional)
Ice cubes (optional)

1 Place all ingredients in a blender and blend until well incorporated.

2 If you prefer a thicker or colder drink, add a few ice cubes and blend again. Serve immediately.

Variation: Use frozen pineapple instead of mango.

GREEN POWER JUICE

TOOLS	TIME	YIELD	DIFFICULTY
	5 MINUTES	2 CUPS	●○○○

1 small pear, cored

4 large leaves kale

½ cup fresh mint leaves, loosely packed

2 large cucumbers, peeled

1 lemon, juiced (about 2 tablespoons)

1 Feed the pear, kale, and mint leaves into a juicer; end with the cucumbers to help ensure that the kale and mint get pushed through.

2 Add the lemon juice, stir, and serve immediately.

Variation: Substitute apple for the pear, or for a less-sweet version, use celery instead of pear.

GINGER BOOST JUICE

TOOLS	TIME	YIELD	DIFFICULTY
	5 MINUTES	2 CUPS	●○○○

1 large cucumber, peeled

3 ribs celery

½ cup parsley leaves, loosely packed

1-inch piece ginger, peeled

2 medium carrots, peeled

1 Feed the cucumber, celery, parsley, and ginger into a juicer; end with the carrots to help push all the ingredients through. Stir and serve immediately.

Variation: Substitute half of a beet for the carrots.

INFUSED WATER

TOOLS	TIME	YIELD	DIFFICULTY
	12 HOURS	1 QUART	●○○○

Acidic Fruit:

Lemon
Lime
Grapefruit
Orange

Sweet Fruit/Vegetable:

Blueberry
Raspberry
Peach
Mango
Pineapple
Cherry
Cucumber

Herb:

Mint
Lavender
Sage
Rosemary
Thyme

1 Add a slice of acidic fruit, a handful of sweet fruit or vegetable, and a couple sprigs of your herb to a quart of filtered water.

2 Let sit overnight in the refrigerator. (You can enjoy the infused water immediately, but the longer you let the fruit and herbs infuse the water, the more the flavor will intensify.)

3 Serve and enjoy!

Note: Feel free to use fresh or frozen fruit for this recipe. Also, don't be afraid to try some things I have not listed here – these are my favorites, but the sky is the limit to how many herb and fruit combinations you can come up with!

Storage: Keeps in the refrigerator for several days.

DRESSINGS + SAUCES

CITRUS-AVOCADO DRESSING

TOOLS	TIME	YIELD	DIFFICULTY
	5 MINUTES	1½ CUPS	●○○○

1 avocado, pitted and skinned
Juice of one orange
   (about 1/3 cup)
Juice of one lemon
   (about 2 tablespoons)
¼ cup extra-virgin olive oil
¼ cup filtered water,
   plus more as needed
1 teaspoon apple cider vinegar
¼ teaspoon ginger powder
¼ teaspoon sea salt

1 Combine all ingredients in a blender and mix until well incorporated.

2 If dressing is too thick, add water one tablespoon at a time until desired consistency is reached.

Storage: Keeps for a day, sealed, in the refrigerator.

OLIVE-AVOCADO DRESSING

TOOLS	TIME	YIELD	DIFFICULTY
	5 MINUTES	1 CUP	●○○○

1 avocado, pitted and skinned
⅓ cup extra-virgin olive oil
⅓ cup filtered water
2 teaspoons apple cider vinegar
½ lemon, juiced
   (about 1 tablespoon)
¼ teaspoon sea salt

1 Combine all ingredients in a blender and mix for a few seconds until well incorporated

2 If dressing is too thick, add water one tablespoon at a time until desired consistency is reached.

Storage: Keeps for a day, sealed, in the refrigerator.

RASPBERRY VINAIGRETTE

TOOLS	TIME	YIELD	DIFFICULTY
	5 MINUTES	¾ CUP	●○○○

½ cup extra-virgin olive oil

¼ cup raspberries
(fresh or frozen)

2 tablespoons apple cider vinegar

¼ teaspoon ginger powder

¼ teaspoon sea salt

1 Combine all ingredients in a blender and mix for a few seconds until well incorporated.

Variation: Feel free to use other fruit instead of the raspberries here–plums or figs would be wonderful substitutions.

Storage: Keeps well in the refrigerator for several days. Shake or stir before using.

BLOOD ORANGE VINAIGRETTE

TOOLS	TIME	YIELD	DIFFICULTY
	5 MINUTES	¾ CUP	●○○○

2 blood oranges, juiced
(about ⅓ cup)

½ cup extra-virgin olive oil

2 teaspoons ume plum vinegar

¼ teaspoon ginger powder

1 Combine all the ingredients in a small bowl and whisk to incorporate.

Variation: Use apple cider or coconut vinegars instead of ume plum; but if you do, make sure to add sea salt to taste, as those vinegars are not as salty as the plum. Regular oranges also work well if you can't find blood oranges.

Storage: Keeps for several days, sealed, in the refrigerator.

CAESAR SALAD DRESSING

TOOLS	TIME	YIELD	DIFFICULTY
	5 MINUTES	1 CUP	●○○○

¼ cup Coconut Concentrate (page 45)*

½ cup filtered water or coconut milk

⅓ cup extra-virgin olive oil

2 cloves garlic

1 lemon, juiced (about 2 tablespoons)

¼ teaspoon sea salt

2 anchovy fillets

1 Combine all ingredients in a blender and mix for a minute until well incorporated.

2 If the dressing is too thick, add water one tablespoon at a time until desired consistency is reached.

*Note: In order to measure the coconut concentrate, it is best to soften it in a warm water bath before use as it is solid at room temperature.

Storage: This dressing keeps in the refrigerator for several days, but it will need to be brought to room temperature or slightly warmed before using, as it hardens when chilled.

GINGER-LIME COCONUT CREAM DRESSING

TOOLS	TIME	YIELD	DIFFICULTY
	15 MINUTES	1 CUP	●○○○

½ cup Coconut Concentrate (page 45)*

½ cup filtered water

2 limes, juiced (about 1 tablespoon)

1 teaspoon apple cider vinegar

1 ½ teaspoons minced ginger

¼ teaspoon sea salt

1 Combine all ingredients in a blender and mix for a minute until well incorporated.

2 If the dressing is too thick, add water one tablespoon at a time until desired consistency is reached.

*Note: In order to measure the coconut concentrate, it is best to soften it in a warm water bath before use as it is solid at room temperature.

Storage: This dressing keeps in the refrigerator for several days, but it will need to be brought to room temperature or slightly warmed before using, as it hardens when chilled.

APPLE CIDER VINAIGRETTE

TOOLS	TIME	YIELD	DIFFICULTY
	5 MINUTES	½ CUP	●○○○

½ cup extra-virgin olive oil

2 tablespoons apple cider vinegar

¼ teaspoon ginger powder

¼ teaspoon sea salt

1 Combine the olive oil, vinegar, ginger powder, and salt in a small bowl and whisk to incorporate.

Variation: This is a great basic vinaigrette recipe that adapts well to improvisation; you can add different fruits or herbs as you prefer. Try adding berries, stone fruit, or various fresh herbs to create your own seasonal dressings.

Storage: Keeps well in the refrigerator for several days. Shake or stir before using.

GINGER PLUM VINAIGRETTE

TOOLS	TIME	YIELD	DIFFICULTY
	5 MINUTES	¾ CUP	●○○○

½ cup extra-virgin olive oil

1 tablespoon ume plum vinegar

1 lemon, juiced (about 2 tablespoons)

1 teaspoon ginger powder

1 Combine the olive oil, vinegar, lemon juice, and ginger powder in a small bowl and whisk to incorporate.

Variation: Use apple cider or coconut vinegar instead of ume plum—but if you do, make sure to add sea salt to taste, as those vinegars are not as salty as the plum.

Storage: Keeps well in the refrigerator for several days. Shake or stir before using.

"RANCH" DRESSING

TOOLS	TIME	YIELD	DIFFICULTY
	15 MINUTES	1 CUP	●○○○

¼ cup Coconut Concentrate
(page 45)*

¼ cup extra-virgin olive oil

½ cup filtered water or Creamy
Coconut Milk (page 46)

½ lemon, juiced
(about 1 tablespoon)

1 teaspoon apple cider vinegar

1 clove garlic

1 tablespoon chopped fresh dill

¼ teaspoon sea salt

1 Place all ingredients in a blender and mix until thoroughly combined.

2 If the dressing is too thick, thin it with water until the desired consistency is reached.

*Note: In order to measure the coconut concentrate, it is best to soften it in a warm water bath before use as it is solid at room temperature.

Storage: This dressing keeps in the refrigerator for several days, but it will need to be brought to room temperature or slightly warmed before using, as it hardens when chilled.

COCONUT-BASIL PESTO

TOOLS	TIME	YIELD	DIFFICULTY
	15 MINUTES	1½ CUPS	●○○○

½ cup coconut water or
filtered water

2 cups fresh basil leaves,
tightly packed

¼ cup extra-virgin olive oil

1 ½-inch piece ginger, peeled
and chopped

2 to 3 cloves garlic, chopped

1 tablespoon ume plum
vinegar

1 lemon, juiced
(about 2 tablespoons)

A few sprigs of fresh mint

1 Place all ingredients into a blender and blend on high for 15 seconds, stopping to scrape the sides if needed. If you want a smoother pesto, continue to blend until desired consistency is reached.

Variation: Use apple cider or coconut vinegars and add sea salt to taste, as those vinegars are not as salty as the plum.

Storage: Keeps for a couple of days, sealed, in the refrigerator.

Serving Suggestions: Rainbow Roasted Root Vegetables (page 188), Sautéed Market Greens (page 183)

GARLIC "MAYO"

TOOLS	TIME	YIELD	DIFFICULTY
	15 MINUTES	1½ CUPS	●○○○

½ cup Coconut Concentrate
   (page 45)*

½ cup filtered water, warm

¼ cup extra-virgin olive oil

3 to 4 cloves garlic

¼ teaspoon salt

1 Place all of the ingredients in a blender and blend on high for a minute or two, until a thick sauce forms (when freshly made, it should resemble the consistency of conventional mayonnaise).

2 If the sauce is too thick, thin with water until the desired consistency is reached.

*Note: In order to measure the coconut concentrate, it is best to soften it in a warm water bath before use as it is solid at room temperature.

Storage: Keeps well in the refrigerator, but hardens. Let come to room temperature or warm to soften before using.

Serving Suggestions: Use to create dressings and sauces, as a topping for Three-Herb Beef Patties (page 262) or Garlic-Sage Chicken Patties (page 211), or as a dip for Rainbow Root Vegetable Chips (page 95)

GUACAMOLE

TOOLS	TIME	YIELD	DIFFICULTY
	15 MINUTES	2 CUPS	●○○○

2 large avocados, pitted and
mashed

½ cup finely chopped
cucumber

¼ cup minced red onion

¼ cup chopped cilantro

1 clove garlic, minced

1 lime, juiced
(about ½ tablespoon)

1 tablespoon extra-virgin
olive oil

1 ½ teaspoons apple cider
vinegar

Sea salt

1 Combine all ingredients in a bowl and stir to combine. Season to taste with salt. Serve Immediately.

Storage: Keeps for a day in the refrigerator

Serving Suggestions: Serve on fresh vegetable slices, Rainbow Root Vegetable Chips (page 95), or as a condiment.

MANGO SALSA

TOOLS	TIME	YIELD	DIFFICULTY
	15 MINUTES	2 CUPS	●○○○

1 large mango, peeled and diced

1 avocado, diced

½ small red onion, diced

1 cucumber, diced

1 bunch cilantro, chopped

2 cloves garlic, minced

1/2 teaspoon sea salt

1 tablespoon olive oil

1 lime, juiced
   (about ½ tablespoon)

1 Combine all of the ingredients in a bowl and mix to incorporate.

Variation: Try substituting peaches, basil, and lemon juice for the mango, cilantro, and lime juice.

Storage: Keeps in the refrigerator for several days.

Serving Suggestions: Serve on lettuce boats with Shredded Roast Beef (page 261), Coconut-Crusted Cod (page 241), on top of salads, or as a condiment.

CHERRY BBQ SAUCE

TOOLS	TIME	YIELD	DIFFICULTY
	45 MINUTES	3 CUPS	●●○○

2 tablespoons solid
  cooking fat

1 small yellow onion, chopped

6 cloves garlic, minced

3 cups pitted cherries, fresh
  or frozen, halved

¼ cup maple syrup

3 tablespoons apple cider
  vinegar

1 teaspoon smoked sea salt

1 Heat the solid cooking fat in a saucepan on medium heat. When the fat has melted and the pan is hot, add the onion and cook for 5 minutes. Add the garlic and cook for another couple of minutes, stirring, until fragrant. Add the cherries, maple syrup, cider vinegar, and smoked sea salt.

2 Cook uncovered over low heat for about 30 minutes, or until the mixture thickens considerably. Transfer to a blender and blend on high until smooth.

Variation: Feel free to use plums instead of cherries.

Storage: Keeps in the refrigerator for a week. Also freezes well.

Serving Suggestions: Lemon-Garlic Marinated Chicken (page 219), Herbed Dry-Rub Steak (page 265), Three-Herb Beef Patties (page 262), or instead of Garlic "Mayo" on Portobello Burgers (page 274)

NOMATO SAUCE

TOOLS	TIME	YIELD	DIFFICULTY
	1 HOUR	6 SERVINGS	●●○○

1 tablespoon solid cooking fat

1 large yellow onion, chopped

4 cloves garlic, minced

2 medium beets, chopped

2 medium carrots, chopped

1 tablespoon fresh thyme

1 tablespoon fresh rosemary

1 cup Bone Broth (page 34)

1 teaspoon sea salt

¼ cup chopped fresh basil

1 Heat the cooking fat in a heavy-bottomed pot on medium heat. When the fat has melted and the pan is hot, add the onion and cook for about 5 minutes. Add the garlic and cook for another couple of minutes, stirring. Add the beets, carrots, thyme, and rosemary and cook for another couple of minutes.

2 Add the bone broth and salt; bring to a boil. Lower the heat, then cover and simmer on low for 30 minutes, or until the vegetables are soft.

3 Carefully transfer the mixture to a blender and purée.

4 Add back to the pot and stir in the fresh basil, turning on the heat to cook for 5 more minutes.

Variation: Make this a meat sauce by adding a pound of browned ground beef, lamb, or pork just before adding the basil and simmering for another 10 minutes.

Storage: Keeps in the refrigerator for several days. Also freezes well.

Serving Suggestions: Serve on top of cooked spaghetti squash or zucchini noodles. You can also add Three-Herb Meatballs (page 262) or Lamb Meatballs (page 277) to the sauce.

SALADS

EMERALD KALE SALAD

TOOLS | TIME | YIELD | DIFFICULTY

15 MINUTES | SERVINGS

1 bunch curly-leafed kale,
   stemmed and finely chopped

2 tablespoons olive oil

1 teaspoon sea salt

½ lemon, juiced (1 tablespoon)

¼ cup minced red onion

¼ cup finely chopped
   cucumber

1 Place the chopped kale in a large bowl; drizzle with olive oil and sprinkle with sea salt.

2 Massage the kale gently with your hands for 5 to 10 minutes, until the tough fibers of the kale break down and soften somewhat.

3 Toss with the lemon juice, red onion and cucumber.

Storage: Keeps well in the refrigerator for several days.

Serving Suggestions: Mediterranean Salmon Salad (page 153), Garlic-Sage Chicken Patties (page 211), Curried Chicken Salad (page 224), Herb-Stuffed Trout (page 253), Three-Herb Beef Patties (page 262)

CUCUMBER-MINT SALAD

TOOLS   TIME   YIELD   DIFFICULTY

15 MINUTES   2 SERVINGS   ●○○○

2 large cucumbers, chopped

½ small red onion, thinly sliced

2 tablespoons chopped fresh parsley

2 tablespoons chopped fresh mint

2 tablespoons apple cider vinegar

3 tablespoons extra-virgin olive oil

Sea salt to taste

1 Combine the cucumbers, onion, parsley, and mint in a bowl.

2 In a small bowl, whisk the apple cider vinegar, olive oil, and sea salt.

3 Toss the dressing with the vegetables and serve.

Storage: Keep dressing separate and toss this salad right before serving.

Serving Suggestions: Mediterranean Salmon Salad (page 153), Rosemary-Mint Lamb Patties (page 269), Lamb Chops with Rosemary-Plum Sauce (page 281), Radish and Jicama Tabbouli (page 142)

RADISH AND JICAMA TABBOULI

TOOLS | TIME | YIELD | DIFFICULTY

15 MINUTES

4 SERVINGS

●○○○

1 bunch parsley, chopped

1 bunch radishes, finely chopped

½ pound jicama (about ½ small), peeled and finely chopped

2 carrots, finely chopped

1 cucumber, finely chopped

8 kalamata olives, minced

1 tablespoon minced fresh mint

¼ cup extra-virgin olive oil

2 tablespoons apple cider vinegar

½ lemon, juiced (about 1 tablespoon)

Sea salt to taste

1 Combine the parsley, radishes, jicama, carrots, cucumber, olives, and mint in a large bowl.

2 In a small bowl, whisk the olive oil, vinegar, lemon juice, and salt.

3 Toss the dressing with the salad and serve.

Storage: Keeps in the refrigerator for several days.

Serving Suggestions: Cucumber-Mint Salad (page 141), Rosemary-Mint Lamb Patties (page 269), Mediterranean Salmon (page 242), Salmon Salad with Olives and Cucumber (page 238), Curried Chicken Salad (page 224), Citrus-Ginger Marinated Salmon (page 237)

CABBAGE SLAW WITH OLIVE-AVOCADO DRESSING

TOOLS	TIME	YIELD	DIFFICULTY
	15 MINUTES	4 SERVINGS	●○○○

1 small head Savoy cabbage, chopped (or substitute green or Napa cabbage)

1 small red onion, thinly sliced

3 carrots, grated (about 2 cups)

1 handful chopped fresh parsley

1 cup Olive-Avocado Dressing (page 115)

1 In a large bowl, combine the cabbage, onion, carrots, and most of the parsley.

2 Toss with the vegetables with the dressing and garnish with the remainder of the parsley.

Storage: Keep dressing separate and toss right before serving.

Serving Suggestions: Orange-Rosemary Duck (page 220), Coconut-Crusted Cod (page 241), Shredded Roast Beef (page 261), Citrus-Thyme Pot Roast (page 266)

POMEGRANATE AND ARUGULA
SALAD WITH FENNEL

TOOLS	TIME	YIELD	DIFFICULTY
	15 MINUTES	4 SERVINGS	●○○○

4 cups arugula, loosely packed

1 small fennel bulb, thinly
    sliced

1 cup pomegranate seeds

¼ cup Blood Orange
    Vinaigrette (page 116)

1 Combine the arugula, fennel slices, and pomegranate seeds in a large bowl.

2 Toss with the vinaigrette and serve.

Variation: Substitute Apple Cider Vinaigrette (page 120) for a less sweet variation.

Storage: Keep dressing separate and toss right before serving.

Serving Suggestions: Coconut-Crusted Cod (page 241), Sear-Roasted Halibut (page 246), Citrus-Ginger Marinated Salmon (page 237)

MARKET SALAD

TOOLS	TIME	YIELD	DIFFICULTY
	15 MINUTES	4 SERVINGS	●○○○

1 head butter lettuce, washed
    and leaves separated and torn

½ small red onion, thinly sliced

2 medium carrots, shredded

1 small beet, shredded

1 cucumber, thinly sliced

½ cup button mushrooms, thinly
    sliced

1 cup of vinaigrette (Apple Cider,
    page 120; Ginger-Plum, page
    120; or Blood Orange,
    page 116)

1 avocado, cubed

1 Combine the lettuce, onion, carrots, beet, cucumber, and mushrooms in a large bowl.

2 Add your choice of vinaigrette to the salad and toss gently.

3 Top with fresh avocado and serve.

Storage: Keep dressing separate; toss (and add avocado) right before serving

Serving Suggestions: Curried Chicken Salad (page 224), Mushroom-Stuffed Cornish Hens (page 223), Citrus-Ginger Marinated Salmon (page 237), Sole Fillet with Tarragon-Caper Sauce (page 245), Three-Herb Beef Patties (page 262)

CITRUS-SPINACH SALAD

TOOLS	TIME	YIELD	DIFFICULTY
	15 MINUTES	4 SERVINGS	●○○○

1 large bunch spinach, washed
  and stemmed

2 medium carrots, grated

10 kalamata olives, pitted and
  halved

½ cucumber, chopped

1 cup Citrus-Avocado Dressing
  (page 115)

1 Place the spinach, carrots, olives, and cucumber in a large bowl.

2 Add the dressing and toss to combine.

Storage: Keep dressing separate and toss right before serving.

Serving Suggestions: Orange-Rosemary Duck (page 220), Mushroom-Stuffed Cornish Hens (page 223), Coconut-Crusted Cod (page 241), Sear-Roasted Halibut (page 246)

MEDITERRANEAN SALMON SALAD

TOOLS	TIME	YIELD	DIFFICULTY
	15 MINUTES	2 SERVINGS	●○○○

1 (7-ounce) can BPA-free salmon, drained

2 medium carrots, finely chopped

½ cucumber, finely chopped

10 kalamata olives, pitted and halved

1 tablespoon chopped parsley

3 tablespoons extra-virgin olive oil

Sea salt

1 Place the drained salmon in a small bowl and mash slightly to break it up.

2 Add the carrots, cucumber, olives, parsley, olive oil, and salt to taste. Toss gently to combine.

Storage: Keeps in the refrigerator for several days.

Serving Suggestions: Emerald Kale Salad (page 138), Cucumber-Mint Salad (page 141), Radish and Jicama Tabbouli (page 142), Market Salad (page 149)

CHICKEN CAESAR SALAD

TOOLS   TIME   YIELD   DIFFICULTY

4

15 MINUTES   SERVINGS   ●●○○

1 large head romaine lettuce, chopped

1 bunch radishes, thinly sliced

2 pounds shredded chicken breast (page 212)

1 cup Caesar Salad Dressing, room temperature (page 119)

1 avocado, cubed (optional)

1 Place the lettuce, radishes, shredded chicken, and dressing in a large bowl and toss well to combine.

2 Add the avocado and serve immediately.

Storage: Keep dressing separate; toss (and add avocado) right before serving.

Serving Suggestions: Rainbow Roasted Root Vegetables (page 188), Rosemary-Roasted Carrots and Parsnips (page 203), Roasted Mixed Vegetables (page 199)

SEARED AHI TUNA SALAD WITH CITRUS-AVOCADO DRESSING

TOOLS | TIME | YIELD | DIFFICULTY

20 MINUTES | 4 SERVINGS

4 (6-ounce) ahi tuna steaks, at room temperature

¼ teaspoon sea salt

1 tablespoon coconut oil

1 large head romaine, shredded

1 carrot, grated

1 cucumber, halved and sliced thinly

1 avocado, cubed

1 tangerine, sectioned

1 cup Citrus-Avocado Dressing (page 115)

1 Salt the tuna on both sides.

2 Heat the coconut oil in a skillet on medium-high heat until lightly smoking.

3 Sear the tuna for about 1 1/2 minutes per side (for medium rare), or until it reaches your desired doneness. Remove from heat, slice thinly, and set aside.

4 Place the romaine, grated carrot, and cucumber in a bowl and toss to combine.

5 Divide the lettuce mixture between several plates; add portions of seared tuna, avocado cubes, and tangerine slices. Serve with dressing poured over the top.

Storage: Serve this salad the day you make it.

SOUPS + STEWS

BEEF-BUTTERNUT STEW WITH PEAR AND THYME

TOOLS	TIME	YIELD	DIFFICULTY
	2 HOURS + 15 MINUTES	6 SERVINGS	●●●○

2 tablespoons solid cooking fat

2 to 3 pounds pastured beef stew meat, cut into 1 ½-inch cubes

1 large yellow onion, chopped

5 cloves garlic, minced

2-inch piece ginger, peeled and minced

2 cups Bone Broth (page 34)

1 bay leaf

1 small butternut squash, peeled and cubed

½ teaspoon cinnamon

½ teaspoon sea salt

2 firm pears, peeled and chopped

1 cup sliced mushrooms, for garnish

1 tablespoon chopped fresh thyme, for garnish

1 Heat 1 tablespoon of the cooking fat in a heavy-bottomed pot on medium-high heat.

2 When the fat has melted and the pan is hot, brown the meat in batches. Remove from the pot, and turn the heat down to medium.

3 Add the onions and cook for about 5 minutes, stirring, until they begin to soften. Add the ginger and garlic, and cook for another couple of minutes, being careful to stir them so that they don't burn.

4 Return the meat to the pot, add the bone broth and bay leaf, and bring to a boil. Immediately turn down to a bare simmer. Cover tightly and cook for 45 minutes.

5 Add the butternut squash, cinnamon, and salt and continue to simmer, covered, for another 15 minutes.

6 Add the pears and simmer for another 30 minutes, or until the meat and squash are both tender.

7 In a small skillet, heat the rest of the cooking fat on medium-high heat and sauté the mushrooms for about 5 minutes, or until they are soft and have browned slightly.

8 Remove the bay leaf. Serve the stew in bowls, garnished with the sautéed mushrooms and a sprinkle of fresh thyme.

Storage: Keeps well in the refrigerator for several days; also freezes well.

BEET AND FENNEL SOUP

TOOLS

TIME
1 HOUR
30 MINUTES

YIELD
4
SERVINGS

DIFFICULTY
●●○○

2 tablespoons solid cooking fat
1 large fennel bulb, ends removed, thinly sliced
2 cloves garlic, minced
1-inch piece ginger, peeled and minced
3 cups Bone Broth (page 34)
2 pounds beets (about 3 medium), peeled and cut into 1½-inch chunks
1 bay leaf
1 teaspoon sea salt
½ lemon, juiced (about 1 tablespoon)
Fennel fronds, for garnish

1 In a heavy-bottomed pot, heat the cooking fat on medium heat. When the fat has melted and the pan is hot, sauté the fennel for about 10 minutes, or until it softens. Add the garlic and ginger to the pot and cook for a few more minutes, stirring.

2 Add the broth, beets, bay leaf, and salt. Bring to a boil, cover, then turn down to a simmer. Cook for 1 hour and 15 minutes, or until the beets are very tender.

3 Remove the bay leaf. Carefully transfer the soup to a high-powered blender or food processor. Blend until desired consistency is reached, adding more broth if needed. Serve warm, with a squeeze of lemon juice and fennel fronds to garnish.

Storage: Keeps well in the refrigerator for several days; also freezes well.

CARROT-GINGER SOUP

TOOLS

TIME
45 MINUTES

YIELD
4
SERVINGS

DIFFICULTY
●●○○

2 tablespoons solid cooking fat
1 small yellow onion, chopped
2-inch piece of ginger, peeled and minced
3 cloves garlic, minced
2 pounds carrots (about 6 medium), chopped
1 tablespoon apple cider vinegar
4 cups Bone Broth (page 34)
1 bay leaf
½ teaspoon cinnamon
1½ teaspoons sea salt
1 tablespoon minced chives, for garnish

1 Heat the cooking fat over medium heat in a heavy-bottomed pot. When the fat has melted and the pan is hot, add the onions, and cook for about 5 minutes, stirring, until they begin to soften. Add the ginger and garlic and cook for a couple more minutes, stirring to ensure that they don't burn. Add the carrots and cook another 10 minutes, stirring often.

2 Add the vinegar, bone broth, bay leaf, cinnamon, and salt to the pot. Bring to a boil, turn down to a gentle simmer and cover tightly with a lid. Cook for 20 minutes, or until carrots are very soft.

3 Turn off the heat, remove the bay leaf and carefully transfer the soup to a high-powered blender or food processor. Purée until the soup reaches your desired thickness, adding more broth if needed. Serve with a sprinkle of chives for garnish.

Storage: Keeps well in the refrigerator for several days; also freezes well.

CLASSIC CHICKEN SOUP

TOOLS | TIME | YIELD | DIFFICULTY

6 SERVINGS

2 HOURS

One 4- to 5-pound stewing hen
   or rooster
1 large onion, chopped
1 bay leaf
2 cloves garlic
1 tablespoon sea salt, plus more
   as needed
6 large carrots, chopped
6 ribs celery, chopped
2 pounds green beans, chopped

1 Begin by cleaning the chicken (rinse it under cold water and remove loose bits of fat and other tissue). Place it in a large stockpot. If it doesn't fit, you will have to cut it into quarters.

2 Add the onion, bay leaf, garlic, and 1 tablespoon salt. Fill the pot with cold water until the chicken is just covered. Bring to a boil, then cover tightly and lower the heat to a bare simmer. Cook this way until the meat is tender and falling off the bone, about 1 to 2 hours—the lower the simmer, the more tender your chicken will come out. Skim the surface of the broth to remove any scum that may appear during cooking.

3 Remove the chicken from the pot and set it aside. Pour the vegetables and broth through a strainer, being careful to save the broth! Discard the vegetables and the bay leaf.

4 Add the broth back to the pot along with the carrots, celery, and green beans. Bring to a boil, then lower the heat. Cover and cook at a simmer for about 20 minutes, or until the vegetables are tender.

5 While the vegetables are cooking, remove the meat from the chicken carcass and set it aside in a bowl.

6 When the veggies are tender, add the chicken back to the soup and simmer for another 20 minutes. Add more salt to taste and serve.

Storage: Keeps well in the refrigerator for several days; also freezes well.

COLD AVOCADO-CUCUMBER SOUP

TOOLS | TIME | YIELD | DIFFICULTY

15 MINUTES | 2 SERVINGS

1 avocado

2 large cucumbers, chopped

¾ cup filtered water

¼ cup extra-virgin olive oil,
 plus more for garnish

2 tablespoons chopped
 fresh mint

1-inch piece ginger, peeled and
 minced

1 clove garlic

½ lemon, juiced
 (about 1 tablespoon)

½ tablespoon apple cider
 vinegar

½ teaspoon sea salt

Fresh mint sprigs, for garnish

Olive oil, for drizzling

1 Make sure all ingredients are well chilled when you begin this recipe so that the finished soup will be cold when served.

3 Cut the avocado in half, then pit and peel it. Cut one of the halves into slices and set them aside. Place the other avocado half and all of the remaining ingredients (except the olive oil and mint sprigs) in a high-powered blender and blend on high until perfectly smooth.

3 Serve immediately, topped with the avocado slices, a sprig of mint, and a drizzle of olive oil.

CREAMY CELERIAC AND LEEK SOUP

TOOLS	TIME	YIELD	DIFFICULTY
	45 MINUTES	4 SERVINGS	●●○○

4 slices sugar-free bacon

2 leeks, washed, ends removed, and sliced thinly

3 cloves garlic, minced

1-inch piece ginger, peeled and minced

4 cups Bone Broth (page 34)

2 pounds celeriac (also called celery root), peeled and cut into 1 ½-inch chunks

1 tablespoon apple cider vinegar

½ teaspoon sea salt

1 bay leaf

A few sprigs of parsley, for garnish

1 Add the bacon to a heavy-bottomed pot over medium heat. Cook until crispy, flipping as needed. Remove the bacon to cool, leaving the fat in the bottom of the pan.

2 Add the leeks and cook for 5 minutes, stirring. Add the garlic and ginger and cook, stirring, for another couple of minutes.

3 Add the broth, celeriac, vinegar, salt, and bay leaf and bring to a boil. Turn down to a simmer, cover, and cook for 15 minutes, or until celeriac is soft.

4 While the soup is cooking, crumble the bacon into small bits.

5 Remove the bay leaf, transfer to a blender and process until desired consistency is reached, adding more broth if needed.

6 Serve garnished with parsley and crumbled bacon on top.

Storage: Keeps well in the refrigerator for several days; also freezes well.

WINTER SQUASH SOUP

TOOLS | TIME | YIELD | DIFFICULTY

1 HOUR 30 MINUTES

6 SERVINGS

●●○○

4 pounds kabocha squash, halved, seeds removed

3 tablespoons solid cooking fat

1 onion, chopped

4 cloves garlic, minced

2 cups Bone Broth (page 34), plus more as needed

1 teaspoon sea salt

1 teaspoon cinnamon

Sliced avocado, for garnish

Chopped fresh parsley, for garnish

1 Preheat the oven to 400 degrees F.

2 Place the squash cut-side up in a baking dish. Spread 2 tablespoons of the cooking fat all over the flesh of the squash and on the bottom of the pan. Bake for 1 hour, or until completely tender.

3 While the squash is baking, heat the remaining tablespoon of the cooking fat in a large, heavy-bottomed pot. Cook the onion for about 10 minutes, stirring, and then add the garlic for a couple of minutes, stirring. Set aside.

4 Remove the squash from the oven and allow it to cool enough to handle. Scoop out the flesh and blend in batches with the onion mixture, bone broth, salt, and cinnamon. If the soup is too thick, add more broth or water, ¼ cup at a time, until desired consistency is reached.

5 Pour the purée back into the large pot and reheat, adding salt to taste. Serve with slices of avocado and parsley for garnish.

Variation: Feel free to use any other type of hard winter squash for this recipe—butternut, acorn, and pumpkin all work well.

Storage: Keeps well in the refrigerator for several days; also freezes well (both without the avocado).

HEARTY VEGETABLE SOUP

TOOLS	TIME	YIELD	DIFFICULTY
	1 HOUR	**6** SERVINGS	●○○○

1 tablespoon solid cooking fat

1 large yellow onion, chopped

3 cloves garlic, minced

1-inch piece ginger, peeled and
   minced

4 carrots, cut into 1 ½-inch
   chunks

2 parsnips, cut into 1 ½-inch
   chunks

1 large sweet potato, peeled and
   cut into 1 ½-inch chunks

1 cup crimini mushrooms, halved

1 tablespoon chopped rosemary

1 tablespoon chopped thyme

1 tablespoon apple cider vinegar

2 quarts Bone Broth (page 34)

1 bay leaf

1 teaspoon sea salt

1 bunch chard, stemmed and
   chopped

1 Heat the cooking fat in a heavy-bottomed pot over medium-high heat. Add the onion and cook, stirring, for 5 minutes. Add the garlic and ginger; cook for another couple of minutes, stirring. Add the carrots, parsnips, sweet potato, mushrooms, rosemary, and thyme, and sauté for another 5 minutes, or until the outsides of the vegetables are lightly browned.

2 Add the vinegar, bone broth, bay leaf, and salt. Bring to a boil, then reduce the heat, cover, and let the soup simmer gently. Cook for about 20 minutes, or until the vegetables are tender.

3 Add the chard during the last couple minutes of cooking, and let the pieces soften in the warm broth. Check to see that the broth is salty enough; add more if needed. Remove the bay leaf before serving.

Variation: Feel free to switch up the root vegetables in this recipe—turnip and rutabaga are nice choices if they are available. You can also use kale or collard greens instead of the chard.

Storage: Keeps well in the refrigerator for several days; also freezes well.

MOROCCAN LAMB STEW

TOOLS | TIME | YIELD | DIFFICULTY

2 HOURS | 4 SERVINGS | ●●○○

½ teaspoon cinnamon

1 teaspoon sea salt

2 pounds lamb stew meat

2 tablespoons solid cooking fat

1 onion, chopped

4 cloves garlic, minced

2-inch piece ginger, peeled and minced

2 tablespoons minced fresh rosemary

1 tablespoon apple cider vinegar

½ cup Bone Broth (page 34)

½ cup filtered water

4 cups chopped carrots

5 dates, minced

2 small blood oranges, zested and juiced (reserve 1 teaspoon zest)

¼ cup chopped cilantro, for garnish

1 In a small bowl, combine the cinnamon and sea salt, and use it to coat the stew meat.

2 Heat the fat in a heavy-bottomed pot on medium heat. When the fat has melted and the pan is hot, brown the meat in batches. Remove the meat from the pot and set aside. Add the onion and cook for 5 minutes, stirring. Next add the garlic, ginger, and rosemary, and cook another couple of minutes, until fragrant.

3 Add the vinegar, bone broth, water, carrots, dates, and blood-orange juice (you should have about ⅓ cup) to the pot with the lamb; bring to a boil. Turn down to a bare simmer, cover, and cook for about 1 ½ hours, until lamb and veggies are all tender.

4 Stir in the orange zest. Serve garnished with cilantro.

Variation: Feel free to use any other type of red meat in this recipe if you do not have lamb available to you. Also, regular oranges will work well if you cannot find blood oranges.

Storage: Keeps well in the refrigerator for several days; also freezes well.

UNDER THE WEATHER SOUP

TOOLS · TIME · YIELD · DIFFICULTY

1 HOUR

4 QUARTS

●●○○

2 quarts Bone Broth (page 34)

1 quart filtered water

3 medium sweet potatoes

1 teaspoon sea salt

1 pound green beans, roughly chopped

2 zucchini, roughly chopped

1 bunch leafy greens (like kale or chard), stemmed and roughly chopped

4 cloves garlic, peeled and chopped

2-inch piece ginger, peeled and chopped

Juice of 1 lemon (about 2 tablespoons), for finishing

1 avocado, thinly sliced, for garnish

1 Place the bone broth, water, sweet potatoes and salt in a large stockpot and bring to a boil. Turn down to a simmer and cook for 20 to 30 minutes, or until the sweet potatoes are tender.

2 Turn off the heat and add the green beans, zucchini, and leafy greens. Cover and let the soup sit for a few minutes, so that the vegetables soften a little but don't cook. Add the salt, garlic, and ginger.

3 Blend the soup in batches and transfer it to another large pot. Reheat gently.

4 Serve with additional salt as needed, a squeeze of lemon juice, and avocado slices.

Variation: Use winter squash instead of sweet potatoes. You can also replace the quart of water with more bone broth for a super healing variation.

Storage: Keeps well in the refrigerator for several days; also freezes well.

CURRIED CHICKEN AND VEGETABLE SOUP

TOOLS	TIME	YIELD	DIFFICULTY
	1 HOUR	6 SERVINGS	●●○○

1 tablespoon solid cooking fat

1 onion, chopped

4 cloves garlic, minced

1 ½-inch piece ginger, peeled and minced

4 cups Bone Broth (page 34)

2 pounds celery root (celeriac), peeled and cut into 2-inch chunks

1 carrot, cut into thin rounds

1 tablespoon turmeric

1 teaspoon sea salt

1 cup thinly sliced mushrooms,

2 pounds shredded chicken breast meat (see page 212)

2 cups Creamy Coconut Milk (page 46)

1 lime, juiced (about ½ tablespoon)

¼ cup chopped cilantro, for garnish

1 Heat the cooking fat in the bottom of a heavy-bottomed pot on medium. When the fat has melted and the pan is hot, add the onions and cook, stirring, for 5 minutes. Add the garlic and ginger, and cook for another couple of minutes, stirring.

2 Add the bone broth, celery root, carrot, turmeric, and salt to the pot. Bring to a boil, then reduce the heat to low and simmer, covered, for 20 minutes.

3 Remove 2 cups of the soup and purée in a blender. Return the purée to the pot; add the mushrooms and shredded chicken. Simmer for another 10 minutes. Turn off the heat and add the coconut milk.

4 Serve each bowl with a squeeze of lime and a sprinkle of fresh cilantro.

Storage: Keeps well in the refrigerator for several days; also freezes well.

VEGETABLES

SAUTÉED MARKET GREENS

TOOLS | TIME | YIELD | DIFFICULTY

20 MINUTES | 4 SERVINGS | ●○○○

2 large bunches kale, chard, or collard greens, stemmed and roughly chopped
2 tablespoons solid cooking fat
1 teaspoon sea salt

1 Wash and dry the greens thoroughly, making sure they are not too wet before cooking.

2 Heat the cooking fat in a large skillet on medium heat. When the fat has melted and the pan is hot, add the greens in batches, stirring as they cook. It's OK if they don't all fit in the pan at once—just keep adding more of the raw pieces as the others cook down. Add the salt and cook for about 15 minutes, turning, or until tender. Serve warm.

Variation: Feel free to use any varieties of large-leafed brassica vegetables (also known as cruciferous vegetables, cabbages, or mustards) for this recipe.

Storage: Keeps in the refrigerator for several days

Serving Suggestions: Coconut-Basil Pesto (page 124), Roasted Mixed Vegetables (page 199), Cinnamon-Scented Butternut Squash (page 184), Lemon-Garlic Marinated Chicken (page 219), Sage-Braised Chicken Legs (page 228), Orange Duck (page 220), Sear-Roasted Halibut (page 246), Braised Lamb Shanks (page 273), Rosemary Shredded Beef Skillet (page 278)

CINNAMON-SCENTED
BUTTERNUT SQUASH

TOOLS	TIME	YIELD	DIFFICULTY
	1 HOUR 15 MINUTES	**4** SERVINGS	●○○○

3 pounds butternut squash, peeled, seeds removed, and cut into 1 ½-inch cubes

2 tablespoons solid cooking fat, melted

¼ teaspoon cinnamon

⅛ teaspoon ginger powder

¼ teaspoon sea salt

1 Preheat the oven to 400 degrees F.

2 Place the butternut squash in a large bowl and combine with the cooking fat, cinnamon, ginger, and salt, stirring to coat evenly.

3 Place in a baking dish and cook for 1 hour, or until completely tender, making sure to stir every 20 minutes or so. Serve warm.

Variation: Feel free to use any type of winter squash for this recipe–pumpkin, acorn, and kabocha all work well.

Storage: Keeps in the refrigerator for several days.

Serving Suggestions: Sautéed Market Greens (page 183), Rosemary Grilled Asparagus (page 195), Chicken and Pesto Sauté (page 216), Lemon-Garlic Marinated Chicken (page 219), Herbed Roast Chicken (page 227)

CURRIED CAULIFLOWER

TOOLS | TIME | YIELD | DIFFICULTY

20 MINUTES | **4** SERVINGS | ●○○○

2 tablespoons solid cooking fat

1 large head cauliflower, chopped into 1-inch pieces

½ teaspoon turmeric powder

½ teaspoon ginger powder

¼ teaspoon sea salt

1 tablespoon coconut aminos (optional)

1 Heat the fat in a wok or large skillet on medium heat.

2 When the fat has melted and the pan is hot, add the cauliflower and sprinkle with the turmeric, ginger, and salt, stirring to combine. Cover and cook for 10 minutes or until the cauliflower is just tender, stirring a couple of times.

3 Add the coconut aminos and cook for another minute.

Variation: Sauté some minced shallots and garlic before adding the cauliflower.

Storage: Keeps in the refrigerator for several days

Serving Suggestions: Asian-Marinated Grilled Chicken (page 219), Citrus-Ginger Marinated Salmon (page 237), Shrimp and Green Bean Stir-Fry (page 249), Garlic Beef and Broccoli (page 270)

RAINBOW ROASTED ROOT VEGETABLES

TOOLS	TIME	YIELD	DIFFICULTY
	1 HOUR	**4** SERVINGS	●○○○

5 medium carrots, cut into 1-inch pieces

3 medium beets, peeled and cut into 1-inch pieces

3 medium parsnips, peeled and cut into 1-inch pieces

1 small rutabaga, peeled and cut into 1-inch pieces

3 tablespoons solid cooking fat, melted

½ teaspoon sea salt

1 Preheat the oven to 400 degrees F.

2 Combine the carrots, beets, parsnips, and rutabaga in a bowl and coat with the cooking fat and salt.

3 Transfer to a baking dish and bake until soft and browned on the outside, about 1 hour. Make sure to stir a couple of times while cooking. Serve warm.

Note: Feel free to use your own mixture of root vegetables for this recipe, not just the ones called for. Sweet potato, celeriac, and turnips make lovely additions or substitutions to any of the above.

Storage: Keeps in the refrigerator for several days.

Serving Suggestions: Brussels Sprouts with Crispy Bacon (page 191), Sautéed Market Greens (page 183), Seared Broccolini and Basil-Pesto (page 204), Herbed Roast Chicken (page 227), Mushroom-Stuffed Cornish Hens (page 223), Citrus-Ginger Marinated Salmon (page 237), Herb Stuffed Trout (page 253), Cranberry-Braised Beef Short Ribs (page 258)

BRUSSELS SPROUTS
WITH CRISPY BACON

TOOLS　　TIME　　YIELD　　DIFFICULTY

4

30 MINUTES　　SERVINGS

1 ½ **pounds brussels sprouts**
6 slices sugar-free bacon
Sea salt

1 Wash brussels sprouts, cut the stem ends off, slice in half, and set aside.

2 Cook bacon in a skillet over medium heat until crispy, turning as necessary. Remove and set bacon aside to cool, leaving the fat in the pan.

3 Sauté brussels sprouts for about 15 minutes, or until browned on the outside and cooked through.

4 When the bacon has cooled, chop into small bits. Combine with the brussels sprouts and serve warm.

Variation: Substitute any green vegetable for the brussels sprouts, making sure to adjust the cooking time accordingly. Broccoli, kale, chard, or collard greens are all good options.

Storage: Keeps well in the refrigerator for several days, although the bacon loses its crispness.

Serving Suggestions: Garlic-Sage Chicken Patties (page 211), Lemon-Garlic Marinated Chicken (page 219), Cranberry-Braised Beef Short Ribs (page 258), Lamb Chops with Rosemary-Plum Sauce (page 281)

MASHED SWEET POTATOES

TOOLS TIME YIELD DIFFICULTY

1 HOUR

4 SERVINGS

●○○○

1 ½ pounds sweet potatoes (about 2 large), peeled and cubed

1 tablespoon solid cooking fat, melted, plus more as needed

¼ teaspoon sea salt

1 Preheat the oven to 400 degrees F.

2 Combine the sweet potatoes, cooking fat, and salt in a bowl, making sure to coat evenly.

3 Place in a baking dish and cook for 40 minutes or until soft, stirring a couple of times while cooking.

4 Remove from the oven, place in a bowl and mash with a potato masher, adding more fat until desired consistency is reached. Serve warm.

Variation: Feel free to use winter squash instead of sweet potato for this recipe.

Storage: Keeps in the refrigerator for several days.

Serving Suggestions: Sautéed Market Greens (page 183), Rosemary Grilled Asparagus (page 195), Herbed Roast Chicken (page 227), Sage-Braised Chicken Legs (page 228), Mushroom Stuffed Cornish Hens (page 223), Herb-Stuffed Whole Trout (page 253), Citrus-Thyme Pot Roast (page 266)

ROSEMARY GRILLED ASPARAGUS

TOOLS   TIME   YIELD   DIFFICULTY

4

30 MINUTES   SERVINGS

2 pounds asparagus, rinsed and dried, ends trimmed

2 tablespoons solid cooking fat, melted

½ tablespoon minced fresh rosemary

¼ teaspoon sea salt

½ lemon, for finishing

1 Preheat your grill or grill pan.

2 Coat the asparagus evenly with the cooking fat, rosemary, and salt.

3 Grill for 10 minutes or until soft, turning occasionally, removing some of the thinner spears as they cook. Serve warm with a squeeze of fresh lemon juice.

Variation: You can also bake these for 10 to 12 minutes in a 400-degree oven.

Storage: Keeps well in the refrigerator for several days (although the asparagus may turn a duller shade of green due to the acidic properties of the lemon juice).

Serving Suggestions: Rainbow Roasted Root Vegetables (page 188), Lemon-Garlic Marinated Grilled Chicken (page 219), Herbed Roast Chicken (page 227), Citrus-Ginger Salmon (page 237), Herbed Dry-Rub Steak (page 265)

PURÉED PARSNIPS

TOOLS   TIME   YIELD   DIFFICULTY

1 HOUR   **4**   ●●○○

SERVINGS

1 ½ pounds parsnips, peeled and chopped into chunks

2 tablespoons solid cooking fat, melted, plus more as needed

¼ teaspoon sea salt

1 Preheat the oven to 400 degrees F.

2 Place the parsnips in a bowl and toss to coat evenly with the cooking fat and salt.

3 Place in a baking dish and cook in the oven for 1 hour or until soft, stirring a couple of times while cooking.

4 Purée in a high-powered blender or food processor until desired consistency is reached (you may like the puréed parsnips a bit on the chunky side or very smooth), adding more fat if necessary. Serve warm.

Storage: Keeps in the refrigerator for several days.

Serving Suggestions: Brussels Sprouts with Crispy Bacon (page 191), Sage-Braised Chicken Legs (page 228), Cranberry-Braised Beef Short Ribs (page 258), Braised Lamb Shanks (page 273), Lamb Chops (page 281)

ROASTED MIXED VEGETABLES

TOOLS | TIME | YIELD | DIFFICULTY

45 MINUTES

4 SERVINGS

●○○○

1 large onion, peeled and
  quartered

4 zucchini, cut in half lengthwise

2 portobello mushroom caps,
  stemmed and halved

2 tablespoons solid cooking fat,
  melted

1 tablespoon minced fresh
  rosemary

Sea salt to taste

1 Preheat the oven to 400 degrees F.

2 Place the onion, zucchini halves, and mushrooms in a bowl and coat evenly with the cooking fat, rosemary, and salt.

3 Spread on a baking sheet and cook in the oven for 30 minutes or until vegetables are tender and the outsides are caramelized. Serve warm.

Storage: Keeps in the refrigerator for several days.

Serving Suggestions: Chicken and Pesto Sauté (page 216), Herbed Roast Chicken (page 227), Mediterranean Salmon (page 242), Sole Fillet with Tarragon-Caper Sauce (page 245), Herb Stuffed Trout (page 253), Cranberry-Braised Beef Short Ribs (page 258), Braised Lamb Shanks (page 273), "Spaghetti" and Meatballs (page 282)

CAULIFLOWER "FRIED RICE"

TOOLS	TIME	YIELD	DIFFICULTY
	15 MINUTES	4 SERVINGS	●●○○

1 small head cauliflower, cored and roughly chopped

2 tablespoons solid cooking fat

1 small yellow onion, finely chopped

4 cloves garlic, minced

1 carrot, finely chopped

1 zucchini, finely chopped

1 cup mushrooms, finely chopped

¼ teaspoon sea salt

½ teaspoon powdered ginger

½ teaspoon turmeric

1 tablespoon coconut aminos

1 tablespoon chopped chives

1 Process the cauliflower in a food processor for 10 seconds, or until it just barely forms rice-size granules; set aside.

2 Heat the cooking fat in the bottom of a large skillet or wok on medium-high heat. When the fat has melted and the pan is hot, add the onion and cook for 5 minutes, stirring. Add the garlic and cook for a couple of minutes, until fragrant. Add the carrot and zucchini and cook for another 5 minutes, stirring.

3 Add the cauliflower "rice," mushrooms, salt, ginger, turmeric, and coconut aminos, and cook 5 to 10 more minutes, stirring, until the vegetables are all soft. Serve garnished with chives.

Storage: Keeps in the refrigerator for several days.

Serving Suggestions: Asian-Marinated Grilled Chicken (page 219), Chicken Stir-Fry (page 231), Citrus-Ginger Marinated Salmon (page 237), Sear-Roasted Halibut (page 246), Shrimp and Green Bean Stir-Fry (page 249), Garlic Beef and Broccoli (page 270)

ROSEMARY-ROASTED CARROTS AND PARSNIPS

TOOLS	TIME	YIELD	DIFFICULTY
	1 HOUR 15 MINUTES	4 SERVINGS	●○○○

1 pound carrots, ends trimmed, peeled

½ pound parsnips, ends trimmed, peeled

2 tablespoons solid cooking fat, melted

2 tablespoons minced fresh rosemary

Sea salt

1 Preheat the oven to 400 degrees F.

2 Place the carrots and parsnips in a large baking dish; coat evenly with the cooking fat, rosemary, and salt to taste.

3 Cook for about 1 hour, stirring every 20 minutes to ensure even browning. The vegetables are finished when tender and lightly caramelized on the outside.

Storage: Keeps in the refrigerator for several days.

Serving Suggestions: Sautéed Market Greens (page 183), Garlic-Sage Chicken Patties (page 211), Herbed Roast Chicken (page 227), Sage-Braised Chicken Legs (page 228), Stuffed Whole Trout (page 253), Cranberry-Braised Beef Short Ribs (page 258), Citrus-Thyme Pot Roast (page 266)

SEARED BROCCOLINI
WITH COCONUT-BASIL PESTO

TOOLS · TIME · YIELD · DIFFICULTY

30 MINUTES · 4 SERVINGS · ●●○○

2 tablespoons solid cooking fat

4 cups broccolini, washed, ends of stems removed

4 cloves garlic, minced

1 cup Coconut-Basil Pesto (page 124)

1 Heat the cooking fat in a large skillet on high heat. When the fat has melted and the pan is hot, sear the broccolini for a couple of minutes on each side. Turn the heat down to medium, add the garlic and let cook, covered, for about 10 minutes, or until tender.

2 Serve with coconut pesto drizzled over the top.

Storage: Keeps well in the refrigerator.

Serving Suggestions: Curried Cauliflower (page 187), Puréed Parsnips (page 196), Herbed Roast Chicken (page 227)

SWEET POTATO FRIES
WITH GARLIC "MAYO"

TOOLS TIME YIELD DIFFICULTY

45 MINUTES

4 SERVINGS

●●○○

3 large sweet potatoes, peeled and cut into ½ inch-thick fries
¼ cup solid cooking fat, melted
Sea salt
½ cup Garlic "Mayo" (page 127)

1 Preheat the oven to 400 degrees F.

2 Place the sweet potato fries in a large bowl and coat with the cooking fat and salt. Arrange on a series of baking sheets, making sure that the fries have adequate space between them (this is what makes them crispy!). Use 3 to 4 baking sheets if you need to.

3 Bake for 10 minutes, remove from the oven, flip, and bake for another 10 to 15 minutes, watching at the end so that they don't burn.

4 Sprinkle with sea salt to taste and serve with the garlic mayo.

Serving Suggestions: Garlic-Sage Chicken Patties (page 211), Three-Herb Beef Patties (page 262), Portobello Burger (page 274), Cinnamon-Sage Dry Rubbed Steak (page 265)

POULTRY

GARLIC-SAGE
CHICKEN PATTIES

TOOLS	TIME	YIELD	DIFFICULTY
	1 HOUR	6 SERVINGS	●●●○

4 tablespoons solid cooking fat

¼ cup minced onion

4 cloves garlic, minced

3 tablespoons chopped fresh sage

¼ cup plus 1 tablespoon coconut flour, divided

1 teaspoon sea salt

2 pounds pastured chicken thigh meat, ground

1 Heat one tablespoon of the cooking fat in a skillet on medium heat. When the fat has melted and the pan is hot, add the onion and cook for about 5 minutes, stirring, until soft. Add the garlic and sage and continue to cook for a couple of minutes, until the mixture is fragrant.

2 Take the pan off the heat and let the mixture cool. While you are waiting, place the ¼ cup coconut flour on a plate.

3 When the onion mixture is no longer hot, add it to the ground chicken, along with the 1 tablespoon coconut flour and the salt. Mix well, then form into 12 to 14 patties. Dredge them lightly in the coconut flour on the plate.

4 Heat the skillet over medium heat, adding more cooking fat if there isn't any left in the pan. Cook the patties in batches for 10 to 15 minutes per side, until golden brown and completely cooked throughout.

Variation: If you don't want to cook the chicken patties on the stovetop, they can be baked in the oven for about 25 minutes at 400 degrees F. You can also try forming them into meatballs instead of patties. Brown in a skillet with some coconut oil until the meatballs firm up, then add ½ cup of bone broth, cover, and simmer until completely cooked (another 10 minutes or so).

Storage: Keeps in the refrigerator for several days. Also freezes well.

Serving Suggestions: Sautéed Market Greens (page 183), Mashed Sweet Potatoes (page 192), Rosemary Grilled Asparagus (page 195)

SHREDDED CHICKEN BREAST

TOOLS	TIME	YIELD	DIFFICULTY
	30 MINUTES	4 SERVINGS	●●○○

2 pounds pastured chicken
breast, skin on

¼ teaspoon sea salt

2 tablespoons solid cooking fat

1 cup Bone Broth (page 34) or
water

1 Rinse the chicken breasts with cold water and pat dry. Bring to room temperature and sprinkle them with the salt.

2 Heat the cooking fat in a skillet over medium heat.

3 When the fat is melted and the pan is hot, place the chicken top-side down and cook for 5 to 7 minutes, or until browned. Flip the chicken, add the broth, cover, and lower the heat to a simmer. Cook for about 20 minutes, or until the internal temperature reaches 165 degrees.

4 Let cool and shred the meat (you'll have about 4 cups of shredded chicken breast meat for all sorts of wonderful uses!).

Storage: Keeps for several days in the refrigerator.

Serving Suggestions: Serve on lettuce boats or as a salad with Mango Salsa (page 131) and Guacamole (page 128)

CHICKEN LIVER WITH
RAW GARLIC AND THYME

TOOLS	TIME	YIELD	DIFFICULTY
	30 MINUTES	2 SERVINGS	●●○○

1 pound pastured chicken livers

3 tablespoons extra-virgin
 olive oil

1 lemon, juiced
 (about 2 tablespoons)

4 cloves garlic, minced

¼ teaspoon sea salt

Fresh thyme, for garnish

1 Prepare the livers by washing and drying them thoroughly. You want them to be as dry as possible before cooking to make sure they get nice and crispy.

2 Heat a skillet on medium-high, and when it is hot, dry-fry the livers for 3 to 4 minutes before flipping. Cook for another 2 to 3 minutes on the other side. They are done cooking when they are fully brown and no longer pink inside (you can cut one open to check).

3 Remove from the pan and coat with olive oil, raw garlic, salt, and thyme. Serve warm.

Storage: Keeps in the refrigerator for several days.

Serving Suggestions: Sautéed Market Greens (page 183), Rainbow Roasted Root Vegetables (page 188)

CHICKEN AND PESTO SAUTÉ

TOOLS | TIME | YIELD | DIFFICULTY

30 MINUTES

2-3
SERVINGS

●●○○

2 tablespoons solid cooking fat

1 pound broccolini, roughly chopped

2 cups shredded chicken breast meat (see page 212)

1 cup Coconut-Basil Pesto (page 124)

1 Heat the cooking fat in the bottom of a large cast-iron pan or skillet on medium heat. When the fat has melted and the pan is hot, add the broccolini, cover, and cook for 10 to 15 minutes, stirring occasionally.

2 Add the shredded chicken and coconut pesto and stir to combine. Cook for another minute or two until everything is incorporated.

Variation: Feel free to use broccoli if broccolini is not available to you.

Storage: Keeps in the refrigerator for several days.

Serving Suggestions: Serve on a bed of zucchini noodles, cooked spaghetti squash, or with Roast Mixed Vegetables (page 199)

MARINATED GRILLED CHICKEN

TOOLS	TIME	YIELD	DIFFICULTY
	1 HOUR 15 MINUTES	4 SERVINGS	●●○○

1 ½ pounds pastured chicken breast, butterflied

1 tablespoon solid cooking fat

Asian Marinade Variation:

¼ cup coconut aminos

1 orange, juiced (about ⅓ cup)

1-inch piece ginger, peeled and minced

1 clove garlic, minced

¼ teaspoon sea salt

Lemon-Garlic
Marinade Variation:

2 lemons, juiced (about ¼ cup)

2 cloves garlic, minced

2 tablespoons minced fresh parsley

½ teaspoon sea salt

1 Choose which variation of the marinade you are going to make. Combine the ingredients in a blender and blend for 30 seconds.

2 Pour into a bag or container with the chicken and marinate for 1 to 2 hours, turning halfway through if the chicken is not completely covered in the marinade.

3 When it is time to cook the chicken, brush your grill or grill-pan with the cooking fat and heat over medium-high heat.

4 Remove the chicken, pat dry, and discard the remaining marinade. Cook for about 10 minutes per side, or until the chicken is cooked throughout. Alternatively, bake the chicken in the oven at 400 degrees F. for about 30 minutes.

Storage: Keeps in the refrigerator for several days.

Serving Suggestions: Rosemary Grilled Asparagus (page 195), Cauliflower "Fried Rice" (page 200)

ORANGE-ROSEMARY DUCK

TOOLS　　TIME　　YIELD　　DIFFICULTY

4 HOURS　　4 SERVINGS　　●●●●

One 5-pound pastured duck

5 oranges, juiced and strained
(about 1 cup)

2 tablespoons maple syrup

1 tablespoon minced fresh
rosemary

1 teaspoon sea salt

1 Preheat the oven to 275 degrees F.

2 Rinse the duck with cool water and dry it thoroughly. Cut off the excess skin around the cavity and neck, saving it to render later if desired. Cut a cross-hatch pattern through the skin (being careful not to slice the meat underneath) anywhere there is a lot of fat—particularly around the breast, sides, and thighs of the bird. Make sure the slices are about an inch apart from each other. Fold the wings under and, using kitchen twine, truss the legs together. Place the duck breast-side up on a rack set in a shallow roasting pan.

3 Cook the duck for 45 minutes, removing it once halfway through to prick all over with a sharp knife. The goal of the pricking is to make little holes for the fat to drain out of, so do this wherever there is a lot of fat.

4 Turn the duck so that it is breast-side down and cook for another 45 minutes, removing it once more halfway through to prick the fat. If there is a lot of liquid fat in the bottom of the pan, transfer the duck to another pan while you pour the fat into a jar for future use.

5 Remove the duck, prick the fat and cook for another 45 minutes breast-side up, removing another time halfway through to prick the fat.

6 Remove the duck, prick the fat and cook for another 45 minutes breast down, removing another time halfway through to prick the fat. At this point, the bird will have been in the oven for 3 hours. Measure the internal temperature, and if it is not at 165 degrees measured at the inside of the thigh, continue cooking until it reaches that temperature.

7 While the duck is in the oven for the last time, bring the orange juice, maple syrup, rosemary, and salt to a boil in a small saucepan. Reduce the heat to a simmer, and cook for about 20 minutes, until reduced to a thick glaze.

8 Remove the duck, pour the remaining fat into your jar, and turn the oven up to 400 degrees F. Prick the fat one last time. Using a pastry brush, glaze the entire bird with the orange-rosemary mixture. Cook for a final 5 to 10 minutes, breast up, until the glaze turns a deep mahogany brown (watch closely to make sure it doesn't burn).

9 Let the duck rest, loosely covered, for 20 minutes. Carve and serve.

Note: It is best to clean and dry the duck at least a few hours before cooking, if not the day before—store it in the refrigerator, uncovered, to give it plenty of time to dry. This will help ensure the skin comes out nice and crispy. Duck fat is one of the most flavorful fats to cook with, and tastes wonderful with roasted root vegetables. To render the extra fat, cut the pieces of fat and skin into small pieces, and place them in a small saucepan with a couple tablespoons of water. Simmer until all of the water has evaporated, most of the fat has rendered, and the skin is crispy. Strain and pour the fat into a jar for future use.

Storage: Rendered duck fat can be stored in the fridge for a couple of months. Cooked duck keeps for several days in the refrigerator.

Serving Suggestions: Cabbage Slaw with Olive-Avocado Dressing (page 145), Citrus-Spinach Salad (page 150), Carrot-Ginger Soup (page 162), Rainbow Roasted Root Vegetables (page 188), Rosemary-Roasted Carrots and Parsnips (page 203)

MUSHROOM-STUFFED CORNISH HENS

TOOLS	TIME	YIELD	DIFFICULTY
	1 HOUR 15 MINUTES	**2** SERVINGS	●●●○

1 tablespoon solid cooking fat

½ yellow onion, finely chopped

2 cloves garlic, minced

1 cup of cauliflower, riced*

1 cup finely chopped crimini
  mushrooms

1 tablespoons chopped
  fresh thyme

¼ teaspoon sea salt, plus more
for seasoning

1 large sweet potato, cut into
  1½-inch chunks

2 pastured Cornish game hens

½ lemon, juiced
  (about 1 tablespoon)

1 Preheat the oven to 400 degrees F.

2 Heat the cooking fat in a skillet on medium heat. When the fat has melted and the pan is hot, add the onion and cook for 5 minutes, stirring. Add the garlic and cook another couple of minutes, stirring, until fragrant. Add the cauliflower, mushrooms, thyme, and the ¼ teaspoon salt and cook, stirring for another 5 minutes, until softened but not completely cooked yet. Remove from heat and set aside to cool.

3 Lightly salt the sweet potatoes and place them in a small roasting dish.

4 Rinse the hens with cool water and thoroughly dry each one. Sprinkle sea salt inside the cavity and rub it all over the skin. Stuff the cavities with the cauliflower and mushroom mixture along with a squeeze of lemon.

5 Arrange the game hens, breast-side up, on top of the sweet potatoes in the roasting dish. Bake for 1 hour, removing halfway through to rotate the hens so that the legs that were facing the outside are now facing in. Check to ensure they reach an internal temperature of 165 when measured at the thickest portion of the inside of the thigh.

6 Serve one hen per person, on a bed of roasted sweet potatoes.

*Note: To make cauliflower "rice", place the roughly chopped florets into a food processor and process lightly, until rice-size granules form.

Variation: Substitute another variety of starchy vegetable for the sweet potato, such as hard winter squash or parsnips.

Storage: Keeps in the refrigerator for several days.

Serving Suggestions: Market Salad (page 149), Citrus-Spinach Salad (page 150), Brussels Sprouts with Crispy Bacon (page 191), Sautéed Market Greens (page 183)

CURRIED CHICKEN SALAD

TOOLS	TIME	YIELD	DIFFICULTY
	15 MINUTES	3-4 SERVINGS	●●○○

½ cup Garlic "Mayo" (page 127)

1 teaspoon apple cider vinegar

½ lemon, juiced
 (about 1 tablespoon)

2 teaspoons powdered turmeric

1 teaspoon powdered ginger

¼ teaspoon sea salt

2 cups shredded chicken breast
 meat (page 212)

¼ cup chopped red onion

¼ cup raisins

2 tablespoons chopped parsley,
 for garnish

1 Soften the mayo in a warm water bath until it is a liquid.

2 Combine the mayo, vinegar, lemon juice, turmeric, ginger, and salt in a large bowl and whisk to combine.

3 Add the chicken breast, red onion, and raisins. Stir to combine. Serve garnished with chopped parsley.

Storage: Keeps in the refrigerator for several days.

Serving Suggestions: Market Salad (page 149), Citrus-Spinach Salad (page 150), Radish and Jicama Tabbouli (page 142)

HERBED ROAST CHICKEN

TOOLS	TIME	YIELD	DIFFICULTY
	1 HOUR 30 MINUTES	4 SERVINGS	●●○○

One 3 to 4 pound free-range
   chicken

Sea salt

A few sprigs of assorted fresh
   herbs (thyme, rosemary, and
   sage work well)

4 cloves garlic, peeled and halved

1 lemon, quartered

1 Preheat the oven to 400 degrees F.

2 Rinse the chicken with cool water and dry it thoroughly. Rub salt all over the inside and outside of the chicken. Place it breast up on a rack in a roasting pan. Place the sprigs of herbs and the garlic halves under the skin at the neck and the rear of the bird. Fill the cavity with the lemon quarters and any leftover herbs.

3 Cook for 20 minutes, breast up. Flip the chicken over, then cook for another 20 minutes breast-side down. Flip once again and cook for a final 20 minutes breast up. Check the internal temperature (measured at the thickest part of the thigh), and continue cooking if it is less than 165 degrees. Remove from the oven and let the chicken rest, lightly covered, for about 15 minutes before serving.

Note: If you don't have a rack, you can cook the chicken on top of a bed of carrots and celery.

Storage: Keeps in the refrigerator for several days.

Serving Suggestions: Brussels Sprouts with Crispy Bacon (page 191), Rainbow Roasted Root Vegetables (page 188), Puréed Parsnips (page 196), Roasted Mixed Vegetables (page 199), Sautéed Market Greens (page 183)

SAGE-BRAISED CHICKEN LEGS

TOOLS   TIME   YIELD   DIFFICULTY

1 HOUR 15 MINUTES   4 SERVINGS

3 to 4 pastured whole chicken legs, with skin

2 tablespoons solid cooking fat

6 cloves garlic, chopped

2 cups halved button or crimini mushrooms

¼ cup chopped fresh sage

2 tablespoons apple cider vinegar

⅓ cup Bone Broth (page 34)

⅓ cup filtered water

¼ teaspoon sea salt

½ lemon, juiced (about 1 tablespoon)

1 Preheat the oven to 300 degrees F.

2 Rinse the chicken with cool water and pat it dry. Make sure the chicken is at room temperature before frying.

3 Heat the cooking fat in an oven-proof skillet or cast-iron pan on medium-high heat. When the fat has melted and the pan is hot, brown the chicken, skin-side down for 8 minutes, or until golden and crispy. Remove from the pan and set aside.

4 Turn the heat down to medium and add the garlic, stirring while cooking for a minute. Add the mushrooms and sage, cooking for another few minutes while stirring. Turn off the heat, add the apple cider vinegar and return the chicken to the pan, with the crispy browned skin facing up.

5 Add the bone broth, water, and salt, and place the pan in the oven. Cook for 35 to 45 minutes, or until a thermometer placed in the thickest part of the thigh reads 165 degrees.

6 Serve with some of the pan juices and fresh lemon juice squeezed on top.

Storage: Keeps in the refrigerator for several days.

Serving Suggestions: Parsnip Purée (page 196), Mashed Sweet Potatoes (page 192)

CHICKEN STIR-FRY

TOOLS | TIME | YIELD | DIFFICULTY

30 MINUTES | 4 SERVINGS | ●●○○

2 tablespoons solid cooking fat

1 yellow onion, chopped

6 cloves garlic, minced

1 ½-inch piece ginger, peeled and minced

3 large carrots, thinly sliced on the diagonal

1 pound broccoli, chopped

½ teaspoon sea salt

½ cup coconut aminos

2 cups chopped mushrooms

2 cups shredded chicken breast meat (page 212)

½ lemon, juiced (about 1 tablespoon)

1 Heat the cooking fat in a wok or large skillet on medium heat.

2 When the fat has melted and the pan is hot, add the onion and cook for 5 minutes, stirring. Add the garlic and ginger and cook, stirring for another minute. Add the carrots, broccoli, salt, and coconut aminos and cover. Cook for 10 minutes, stirring occasionally. Add the mushrooms and cook for another 5 minutes. The vegetables should be firm yet cooked.

3 Add the chicken and stir to heat throughout. Squeeze with lemon juice and serve warm.

Storage: Keeps in the refrigerator for several days.

Serving Suggestions: Cauliflower Rice (page 200), Curried Cauliflower (page 187), Puréed Parsnips page 196)

SEAFOOD

CLASSIC TUNA SALAD

TOOLS   TIME   YIELD   DIFFICULTY

3-4

15 MINUTES   SERVINGS

¾ cup Garlic "Mayo" (page 127)

3 cans BPA-free canned tuna, drained (about 15 ounces)

1 large carrot, chopped finely

1 stalk celery, chopped finely

3 tablespoons minced red onion

2 tablespoons minced fresh dill

½ lemon, juiced (about 1 tablespoon)

1 teaspoon apple cider vinegar

¼ teaspoon sea salt

Romaine lettuce, shredded or torn, for serving

1 Soften the mayo in a warm water bath until it is a liquid.

2 Combine the tuna, carrot, celery, red onion, dill, mayo, lemon juice, vinegar, and salt in a bowl and mix to combine.

3 Serve on a bed of lettuce or on lettuce boats (whole lettuce leaves).

Storage: Keeps in the refrigerator for several days.

Serving Suggestions: Emerald Kale Salad (page 138), Citrus-Spinach Salad (page 150), Rainbow Roasted Root Vegetables (page 188)

MARINATED SALMON

TOOLS   TIME   YIELD   DIFFICULTY

1 HOUR
15 MINUTES

4
SERVINGS

●●○○

1 ½ pounds wild-caught salmon fillet

Coconut Amino Marinade Variation:

½ cup coconut aminos
1 lemon, juiced (about 2 tablespoons)
1 tablespoon chopped fresh thyme
¼ teaspoon ginger powder
¼ teaspoon sea salt

Citrus-Ginger Marinade Variation:

2 oranges, juiced (about ⅔ cup)
1 tablespoon apple cider vinegar
1 tablespoon coconut aminos (optional)
2 tablespoons chopped fresh mint
1-inch piece ginger, peeled
¼ teaspoon sea salt

1 Place the salmon fillet in a large bag or container for marinating.

2 Choose which variation of marinade you will be making, and place all of the ingredients in a blender and blend for 30 seconds on high. Pour the marinade ingredients into the bag or container with the salmon and let marinate for 1 hour, flipping once or twice if the marinade doesn't completely cover the fish.

3 When you are ready to cook the salmon, preheat the oven to 400 degrees F. Discard the marinade and place the salmon on an oiled baking sheet. Bake for 15 minutes, or until the fish lightly flakes when tested with a fork. The cooking time may vary a bit depending on the thickness of your fish.

Note: If you don't have a blender, mince everything and whisk with the other marinade ingredients.

Storage: Keeps for a couple of days in the refrigerator.

Serving Suggestions: Cauliflower "Fried Rice" (page 200), Curried Cauliflower (page 187), Market Salad (page 149)

SALMON SALAD WITH OLIVES AND CUCUMBER

TOOLS | TIME | YIELD | DIFFICULTY

15 MINUTES | **3** SERVINGS | ●○○○

¾ cup Garlic "Mayo" (page 127)

½ lemon, juiced
(about 1 tablespoon)

2 tablespoons olive oil

1 teaspoon apple cider vinegar

1/4 teaspoon sea salt

15 ounces BPA-free canned
salmon, drained

½ cucumber, finely chopped

10 kalamata olives, pitted and
finely chopped

4 radishes, minced

3 tablespoons minced red onion

2 tablespoons minced parsley

Mixed salad greens

1 Soften the mayo in a warm water bath until it is liquid.

2 Combine the mayo, lemon juice, olive oil, vinegar, and salt in a large bowl.

3 Add the salmon, cucumber, olives, radishes, red onion, and parsley and mix to combine.

4 Serve on a bed of mixed greens or on lettuce boats (whole lettuce leaves).

Storage: Keeps for a couple of days in the refrigerator.

Serving Suggestions: Olive Tapenade (page 91), Parsley-Garlic Dip (page 96), Emerald Kale Salad (page 138), Radish and Jicama Tabbouli (page 142)

COCONUT-CRUSTED COD

TOOLS | TIME | YIELD | DIFFICULTY

45 MINUTES | 4 SERVINGS | ●●●○

1 ½ cups coconut flour

1 ½ teaspoons ginger powder

¼ teaspoon sea salt

2 cups Creamy Coconut Milk (page 46)

1 cup fine shredded coconut flakes (unsweetened)

1 ½ pounds cod fillet, deboned and cut into 2-inch thick strips

2 tablespoons coconut oil

Mango Salsa (page 131)

1 Combine the coconut flour, ginger powder and salt on a plate. Place the coconut milk in one shallow bowl and the shredded coconut in another.

2 Dip the cod strips into the coconut milk, then the coconut flour mixture, back into the coconut milk, and finally back into the shredded coconut, paying special attention to coating the strips evenly.

3 Heat the coconut oil in a skillet on high heat. Sauté the cod strips for about 5 minutes per side (depending on thickness of the fish), or until the top and bottom are nice and browned and the fish is firm.

4 Serve topped with mango salsa.

Note: Once the cod strips are in the pan, try not to fuss with them too much, as the crust may crumble and fall off (most recipes for breaded fish use egg to help the dry ingredients adhere).

Storage: This dish is at its very best served immediately. You may hold it for several days in the refrigerator, but the coating will lose its crispness.

Serving Suggestions: Pomegranate and Arugula Salad with Fennel (page 146), Cabbage Slaw with Olive Avocado Dressing (page 145), Citrus-Spinach Salad (page 150), Rainbow Roasted Root Vegetables (page 188)

MEDITERRANEAN SALMON

TOOLS   TIME   YIELD   DIFFICULTY

40 MINUTES   **4** SERVINGS   ●●○○

1 tablespoon coconut oil

1 ½ pounds wild-caught salmon fillet

½ cup kalamata olives, pitted and minced

¼ cup chopped fresh parsley

½ lemon, juiced (about 1 tablespoon)

¼ teaspoon sea salt

3 tablespoons extra-virgin olive oil

1 Preheat the oven to 400 degrees F.

2 Spread the coconut oil on a baking sheet. Place the salmon on it, skin-side down.

3 Combine the olives, parsley, lemon juice, and salt in a bowl and spread the mixture all over the fillet.

4 Bake for 15 minutes, or until the fish lightly flakes when tested with a fork. The cooking time may vary a bit depending on the thickness of the fish.

5 Drizzle with the olive oil before serving.

Storage: Keeps for a couple of days in the refrigerator.

Serving Suggestions: Parsley-Garlic Dip (page 96), Cucumber-Mint Salad (page 141), Radish and Jicama Tabbouli (page 142)

SOLE FILLET WITH TARRAGON-CAPER SAUCE

TOOLS   TIME   YIELD   DIFFICULTY

4

30 MINUTES   SERVINGS

½ cup Garlic "Mayo," (page 127)

½ lemon, juiced
   (about 1 tablespoon)

¼ cup minced tarragon

2 tablespoons capers

¼ teaspoon sea salt

2 tablespoons solid cooking fat

1 ½ pounds wild-caught sole

1 Soften the mayo in a warm water bath until it is a liquid.

2 Place the mayo, lemon juice, tarragon, capers, and salt in a small bowl; mix until combined. Set aside.

3 Heat the cooking fat in a skillet on high heat. When the fat has melted and the pan is hot, sear the fish for a minute or two a side, depending on the thickness of the fillets.

4 Remove from the heat and spoon the tarragon-caper sauce over top. Serve immediately.

Storage: Keeps for a couple of days in the refrigerator.

Serving Suggestions: Market Salad (page 149), Rainbow Roasted Root Vegetables (page 188)

SEAR-ROASTED HALIBUT

TOOLS	TIME	YIELD	DIFFICULTY
	15 MINUTES	2 SERVINGS	●●○○

½ orange, juiced
  (about 3 tablespoons)
2 tablespoons coconut aminos
½ lemon, juiced
  (about 1 tablespoon)
¼ teaspoon ginger powder
¼ teaspoon sea salt
2 tablespoons coconut flour
12 ounces fresh halibut, skinned,
  deboned, and cut into
  two portions
2 tablespoons coconut oil
Fresh chives, chopped, for
  garnish

1 Preheat the oven to 400 degrees F.

2 Combine the orange juice, coconut aminos, lemon juice, ginger powder, and half of the salt in a small bowl; stir to combine. Place the coconut flour on a plate and set aside.

3 Sprinkle both sides of the fish with the remaining sea salt and dredge in the coconut flour, using your fingers to create a thin, even coating around all sides of the fish.

4 Heat the coconut oil in an oven-safe skillet on high heat. When it is very hot, add the halibut and sear for 2 minutes, or until browned on the bottom. Flip the fish and place the skillet immediately in the oven. Cook for 3 to 5 minutes, depending on the thickness of the fillet. The fish is finished when it is no longer translucent.

5 Serve with the citrus–coconut amino sauce and garnish with the chopped chives.

Storage: Keeps for a couple of days in the refrigerator.

Serving Suggestions: Citrus-Spinach Salad (page 150), Cauliflower "Fried Rice" (page 200), Curried Cauliflower (page 187)

SHRIMP AND GREEN BEAN STIR-FRY

TOOLS | TIME | YIELD | DIFFICULTY

40 MINUTES | **3** SERVINGS | ●●○○

2 tablespoons solid cooking fat

½ onion, halved and thinly sliced

4 cloves garlic, minced

2-inch piece ginger, peeled and minced

2 pounds green beans, stems removed, halved

1 cup thinly sliced crimini mushrooms

2 tablespoons coconut aminos

1 teaspoon honey

1 pound shrimp, peeled, with tails left on

¼ teaspoon sea salt

Fresh parsley, minced, for garnish

1 Heat the cooking fat in a wok or large skillet on medium-high heat. When the fat has melted and the pan is hot, add the onion and cook for five minutes, stirring. Add the garlic and ginger and cook, stirring for another couple of minutes. Add the green beans and cook for 10 minutes (toss and turn them so they cook evenly).

2 Add the mushrooms, coconut aminos, and honey and cook for a few minutes. Add the shrimp and salt and cook until the shrimp is pink throughout, 3 to 4 minutes. Garnish with the parsley and serve immediately.

Storage: Keeps for a couple of days in the refrigerator.

Serving Suggestions: Cauliflower "Fried Rice" (p.200), Curried Cauliflower (p.187), Carrot Ginger Soup (p.162)

SALMON CHOWDER

TOOLS · TIME · YIELD · DIFFICULTY

2 HOURS · **4** SERVINGS · ●●●●

1 salmon carcass–bones, head, and tail

1 quart water

1 bay leaf

2 tablespoons solid cooking fat

1 large onion, chopped

4 cloves garlic, minced

4 parsnips, chopped

3 carrots, chopped

2 ribs celery, chopped

1 tablespoon apple cider vinegar

1 tablespoon chopped fresh thyme

1 ½ teaspoons sea salt

1 ½ pounds salmon fillet, skin and bones removed, cut into 1 ½-inch chunks

1 cup Creamy Coconut Milk (page 46)

½ lemon, juiced (about 1 tablespoon)

3 green onions, thinly sliced

1 To make the broth, place the salmon carcass, water, and bay leaf in a stockpot, bring to a boil, cover, and turn down to a bare simmer. It is essential to cook this at the lowest simmer possible.

2 Remove and discard the carcass and bay leaf. Strain the broth into a large bowl and set it aside.

3 Heat the cooking fat in a heavy-bottomed pot on medium heat. When the fat has melted and the pan is hot, add the onion and cook for 5 minutes, stirring. Add the garlic, and cook for another couple of minutes, until fragrant. Add the parsnips, carrots, and celery; cook another 5 minutes, stirring, until the vegetables are lightly browned.

4 Add the reserved fish broth, vinegar, thyme, and salt to the pot and bring to a boil. Cover and turn down to a bare simmer, and cook for 30 minutes or until the vegetables are tender.

5 Place 2 cups of the soup in a blender, leaving the carrots behind, if possible as not to turn the soup orange. Blend until smooth, then add the purée back to the soup.

6 Add the salmon chunks and coconut milk to the soup and cook for a few minutes, just until the soup is piping hot (do not let the soup boil).

7 Add the lemon juice and serve garnished with green onions.

Note: Tastes best served fresh, but if you must, reheat gently over low heat

HERB-STUFFED TROUT

TOOLS　　TIME　　YIELD　　DIFFICULTY

2

30 MINUTES　　SERVINGS

●●○○

1 tablespoon solid cooking fat

2 whole trout
(about 1 pound each)

½ teaspoon sea salt

1 lemon, sliced into thin rounds

4 whole sprigs of fresh rosemary

4 whole sprigs of fresh thyme

Kitchen twine

1 Preheat the oven to 450 degrees F.

2 Coat the bottom of a baking dish with the cooking fat. Sprinkle the salt all over the inside and outside of the fish, and place them in the dish.

3 Fill the cavity of each fish with a few lemon rounds and a couple large sprigs of the herbs. Using the twine, tie a loop around the middle of the fish so that the contents stay inside. Alternatively, pin the thinnest part of each belly closed, using skewers or toothpicks.

4 Bake for 15 minutes, or until the fish flakes easily when tested with a fork.

5 Serve whole, eating around the bones, herbs, and lemon in the cavity.

Note: If you have someone in your family who is a fisherman/woman, wild trout is much preferred over the commercial farmed variety!

Serving Suggestions: Emerald Kale Salad (page 138), Cinnamon-Scented Butternut Squash (page 184), Puréed Parsnips (page 196), Carrot Ginger Soup (page 162)

CLAM CHOWDER

TOOLS | TIME | YIELD | DIFFICULTY

1 HOUR 15 MINUTES

4 SERVINGS

● ● ● ●

1 tablespoon sea salt

3 pounds steamer clams

1 ½ cups filtered water

4 slices sugar-free bacon

1 small yellow onion, chopped

2 carrots, chopped

5 cloves garlic, minced

1 tablespoon fresh thyme

1 bay leaf

2 pounds celeriac (celery root), peeled and cut into small cubes

1 cup Creamy Coconut Milk (page 46)

3 green onions, sliced thinly, for garnish

1 Add the salt to a bowl of cool water and stir to dissolve. Add the clams, and allow them to soak for 20 minutes.

2 Clean the clams thoroughly with a wire brush or a stiff vegetable brush, discarding any of them that are broken.

3 Bring the filtered water to a boil in a large pot. Add the clams, cover and reduce the heat to a simmer. After about 4 minutes the clams should start opening, and once they do so, pull them out one by one. Continue doing this until the clams have cooked, about another 4 minutes. If there are any that haven't opened at this point, throw them away. Set the clams aside to cool, then strain the clam broth, reserving 1 ½ cups for the soup.

4 In a heavy-bottomed pot, cook the bacon slices until they are crispy, turning as needed. Remove them from the pot, leaving the fat. Add the onion and cook for 5 minutes, then add the carrots, garlic, thyme, and bay leaf and cook, stirring, for 5 more minutes. Add the reserved clam broth and the celeriac, bring to a boil, then cover and simmer for 5 to 10 minutes, or until the celeriac is soft.

5 Remove the clams from their shells and chop the bacon into bits. Set aside.

6 When the celeriac has finished cooking, turn off the heat, remove the bay leaf, and transfer half of the mixture to a blender. Blend until very smooth, then add the purée back to the pot.

7 Stir in the coconut milk, clams, and bacon bits. Garnish with chopped green onions.

Note: Tastes best served fresh, but if you must, reheat gently over low heat.

BEEF + LAMB

CRANBERRY-BRAISED SHORT RIBS

TOOLS	TIME	YIELD	DIFFICULTY
	2 - 3 HOURS	**4** SERVINGS	●●●○

1 tablespoon solid cooking fat

4 pounds grass-fed beef short ribs

1 cup Bone Broth (page 34)

1 cup unsweetened cranberry juice

1 cup fresh cranberries

1 tablespoon apple cider vinegar

1 bay leaf

¼ teaspoon sea salt

2 tablespoons chopped fresh parsley

1 Preheat the oven to 300 degrees F.

2 Heat the fat in a large, heavy-bottomed pot on medium-high heat. Working in batches, brown the ribs well on all sides.

3 Add the bone broth, cranberry juice, cranberries, vinegar, bay leaf, and salt to the pot. The liquid should come up to about one-third of the level of the meat—if any less, add a little bit more broth or water.

4 Making sure that your lid fits tightly, braise for 2 to 3 hours in the oven, checking periodically that the liquid is barely simmering, and that there is enough liquid (you shouldn't have a problem if the lid seals well). It is finished when the meat is falling off the bone.

5 Carefully transfer the short ribs to a plate and cover the meat. Strain the liquid into a large bowl, then pour it into a saucepan, bring it to a boil, and reduce the quantity by about half (you should have about ¾ cup of juice).

6 Serve with some of the juices poured over the ribs and the parsley sprinkled on top.

Storage: Keeps in the refrigerator for several days.

Serving Suggestions: Puréed Parsnips (page 196), Mashed Sweet Potatoes (page 192), Sautéed Market Greens (page 183), Rosemary Grilled Asparagus (page 195)

SHREDDED ROAST BEEF

TOOLS	TIME	YIELD	DIFFICULTY
	3 - 4 HOURS	**6** SERVINGS	●●○○

1 tablespoon solid cooking fat

Sea salt

One 3 to 4 pound beef roast, cut into 2 or 3 big chunks

1 ½ cups Bone Broth (page 34)

1 tablespoon apple cider vinegar

Fresh herbs (thyme, rosemary, sage, and oregano all work great)

1 Preheat the oven to 275 degrees F.

2 Generously apply salt to the roast.

3 Heat the cooking fat in an oven-safe pot on medium-high heat. When the fat has melted and the pan is hot, brown the chunks of beef on all sides. Turn off the heat.

4 Add the bone broth and vinegar to the pot along with the fresh herbs. Ensuring that your lid is on tightly, cook for 3 to 4 hours, checking periodically to make sure there is liquid in the bottom of the pot. The roast is finished cooking when the meat pulls apart easily with a fork.

5 Remove the meat from the pot and let it cool for a couple of minutes. Meanwhile, strain the juice from the pot, pour it into a small saucepan, and bring it to a simmer. Reduce the liquid until the quantity is about 3/4 cup, about 15 minutes.

6 Once the meat has cooled a little bit, shred it into bits using two forks or your hands.

7 Add the reduced pan juice back to the shredded beef and combine.

Storage: Keeps in the refrigerator for several days. Also freezes well.

Serving Suggestions: Serve on lettuce boats or as a salad with Mango Salsa (page 131) and Guacamole (page 128).

THREE-HERB BEEF PATTIES

TOOLS | TIME | YIELD | DIFFICULTY

40 MINUTES | **6** SERVINGS | ●●○○

2 pounds grass-fed ground beef

1 tablespoon finely chopped
fresh rosemary

1 tablespoon finely chopped
fresh thyme

1 tablespoon finely chopped
fresh sage

1 teaspoon sea salt

1 tablespoon solid cooking fat

1 In a large bowl, combine the ground beef, fresh herbs, and salt.

2 Using your hands, form into 12 patties.

3 Heat the cooking fat in a cast-iron skillet on medium heat. Cook the patties for about 5 to 8 minutes per side, until nicely browned on the outside and cooked throughout. (Alternatively, bake the patties in the oven for about 20 minutes at 400 degrees F.)

Storage: Keeps in the refrigerator for several days. Also freezes well.

Variation: Make meatballs and serve with cooked spaghetti squash or zucchini noodles and Coconut-Basil Pesto (page 124) or Nomato Sauce (page 135).

Serving Suggestions: Emerald Kale Salad (page 138), Market Salad (page 149)

DRY-RUBBED STEAK

TOOLS	TIME	YIELD	DIFFICULTY
	20 MINUTES	4 SERVINGS	●●○○

2 pounds grass-fed beef steaks
1 tablespoon coconut oil

Cinnamon-Sage Variation:

1 ½ tablespoons sea salt
¾ tablespoon ground sage
¾ teaspoon cinnamon

Herbed Variation:

1 tablespoon smoked sea salt
1 tablespoon dried rosemary
1 tablespoon dried thyme
½ tablespoon ground sage

1 Choose which variation of the rub you will be making, and combine the salt, herbs, and spices together in a small bowl.

2 Rub the mixture on both sides of the steaks.

3 Heat the coconut oil in a cast-iron skillet on medium-high heat. When the fat has melted and the pan is hot, cook the steaks 5 to 7 minutes per side, or until desired doneness is reached.

Note: This recipe also works fantastically on the grill.

Variation: Try using lamb chops or steaks instead of beef.

Serving Suggestions: Root Vegetable Chips (page 95), Cabbage Slaw with Olive-Avocado Dressing (page 145), Market Salad (page 149), Rosemary Grilled Asparagus (page 195), Sweet Potato Fries with Garlic "Mayo" (page 209)

CITRUS-THYME POT ROAST

TOOLS	TIME	YIELD	DIFFICULTY
	2 - 3 HOURS	**6** SERVINGS	●●○○

1 tablespoon solid cooking fat

2 to 3 pounds grass-fed
  beef roast

¾ cup Bone Broth (page 34)

2 tablespoons apple cider vinegar

1 orange, juiced (about 1/3 cup)

1 bay leaf

1 ½ teaspoons sea salt

3 carrots, cut into 2-inch chunks

2 parsnips, peeled and cut into
  2-inch chunks

2 tablespoons chopped
  fresh thyme

1 Preheat the oven to 300 degrees F.

2 Heat the cooking fat in the bottom of a heavy-bottomed pot on medium-high heat. Brown the roast well on all sides and remove it from the pot.

3 Add the bone broth, cider vinegar, orange juice, bay leaf, and salt to the pot and stir to combine.

4 Place the roast in the pot and surround it with the carrots and parsnips. Sprinkle the thyme all over the roast and the vegetables.

5 Making sure you have a lid that fits properly, braise the roast for 2 to 3 hours in the oven, checking periodically to make sure that it is covered by at least 1/3 liquid (you shouldn't have a problem if the lid seals well). It is finished when the meat is easily pulled apart with a fork.

6 Remove the bay leaf and serve the meat and vegetables with some of the braising liquid.

Variation: Feel free to use cranberry juice instead of orange, or rosemary or sage instead of the thyme.

Storage: Keeps in the refrigerator for several days.

Serving Suggestions: Citrus-Spinach Salad (page 150), Cinnamon-Scented Butternut Squash (page 184), Puréed Parsnips (page 196), Roasted Mixed Vegetables (page 199), Sautéed Market Greens (page 183)

ROSEMARY-MINT
LAMB PATTIES

TOOLS	TIME	YIELD	DIFFICULTY
	40 MINUTES	6 SERVINGS	●●○○

2 pounds ground lamb

2 tablespoons finely chopped fresh mint

1 tablespoon finely chopped fresh rosemary

1 teaspoon sea salt

½ teaspoon lemon zest

1 tablespoon solid cooking fat

1 In a large bowl, combine the ground lamb, mint, rosemary, salt, and lemon zest.

2 Using your hands, form into 12 patties.

3 Heat some of the cooking fat in a cast-iron skillet on medium heat. Cook the patties for 5 to 8 minutes per side, until nicely browned on the outside and cooked throughout. Alternatively, bake the patties in the oven for about 20 minutes at 400 degrees F.

Storage: Keeps in the refrigerator for several days. Also freezes well.

Serving Suggestions: Cucumber-Mint Salad (page 141), Radish and Jicama Tabbouli (page 142), Emerald Kale Salad (page 138)

GARLIC BEEF AND BROCCOLI

TOOLS	TIME	YIELD	DIFFICULTY
	30 MINUTES	4 SERVINGS	●●○○

½ tablespoon solid cooking fat

2 pounds grass-fed beef steaks, cut into ¼-inch-thick slices

5 cloves garlic, minced

1 ½-inch piece ginger, peeled and minced

1 bunch broccoli, chopped

2 tablespoons water or Bone Broth (page 34)

½ cup coconut aminos

½ lemon, juiced (about 1 tablespoon)

¼ teaspoon sea salt

1 Heat the cooking fat in a wok or large skillet on medium-high heat.

2 When the fat has melted and the pan is hot, sauté the steak slices, stirring, 5 to 7 minutes. Remove and set aside.

3 Lower the heat to medium and add the garlic and ginger, stirring and cooking until fragrant, about 1 minute. Add the broccoli and cook for a few minutes, until lightly browned. Add the water, cover, and reduce the heat to medium-low. Cook for about 10 minutes, stirring occasionally, until the broccoli is tender.

4 Add the coconut aminos, lemon juice, salt, and beef slices back to the pan and sauté, tossing to combine, for a minute or two. Serve immediately.

Storage: Keeps in the refrigerator for several days.

Serving Suggestions: Cauliflower "Fried Rice" (page 200), Curried Cauliflower (page 187)

BRAISED LAMB SHANKS
WITH PARSNIP PURÉE

TOOLS   TIME   YIELD   DIFFICULTY

3-4

3 HOURS   SERVINGS

2 tablespoons solid cooking fat

3 to 4 pounds lamb shanks

1 yellow onion, finely chopped

2 carrots, finely chopped

5 cloves garlic, minced

3 tablespoons minced fresh
 rosemary

1 tablespoon apple cider vinegar

1 ½ cups Bone Broth (page 34)

¼ teaspoon sea salt

1 recipe Parsnip Purée (page 196)

Fresh parsley, chopped, for
 garnish

1 Preheat the oven to 300 degrees F.

2 Heat the cooking fat in a heavy-bottomed, oven-safe pot on medium. When the fat has melted and the pan is hot, brown the lamb shanks well on all sides, about 8 minutes. Remove from the pot and set aside.

3 Add the onion, carrots, garlic, and rosemary; cook 5 to 7 minutes, stirring, until lightly browned.

4 Turn off the heat, add the vinegar, bone broth, the salt, and return the shanks to the pot. The liquid should come up one third to one half the level of the shanks. If it is too low, add a little more water or broth. Cover with a tight-fitting lid and cook in the oven for 2 to 3 hours, until the meat is falling off the bone. Uncover the pot for the last 20 minutes of cooking.

5 Serve on a bed of puréed parsnips with some of the pan juices drizzled on top. Garnish with the parsley.

Variation: Serve on a bed of Mashed Sweet Potatoes (page 192) instead of the Parsnips.

Storage: Keeps in the refrigerator for several days.

Serving Suggestions: Sautéed Market Greens (page 183), Brussels Sprouts with Crispy Bacon (page 191), Rosemary Grilled Asparagus (page 195)

PORTOBELLO "BURGER"

TOOLS   TIME   YIELD   DIFFICULTY

30 MINUTES   4 SERVINGS   ●●○○

4 tablespoons Garlic "Mayo" (page 127)

2 tablespoons solid cooking fat, melted

4 portobello mushroom, stemmed

½ yellow onion, sliced into thick rings

Sea salt

4 to 8 leaves soft lettuce (not romaine)

4 Three-Herb Beef Patties (page 262), warmed

1 avocado, sliced

1 Soften the mayo in a warm water bath until it is a liquid.

2 Heat a skillet or grill-pan over medium heat, using half of the cooking fat.

3 Brush the rest on the portobello caps and onion, also sprinkling with sea salt. Add the mushrooms and onions to the pan and cook for 10 to 15 minutes, flipping once, until fully cooked. Turn off the heat and set aside to cool for a few minutes.

4 Grab a leaf or two of lettuce and construct a "burger," using a beef patty, a tablespoon of mayo, some onion rings and a Portobello. Finish with several slices of avocado.

Serving Suggestions: Rainbow Root Vegetable Chips (page 95), Sweet Potato Fries (page 207) and Garlic "Mayo" (page 127)

LAMB MEATBALLS WITH GARLIC AND SPINACH

TOOLS | TIME | YIELD | DIFFICULTY

3-4

30 MINUTES | SERVINGS

6 kalamata olives, minced

3 cloves garlic, minced

½ teaspoon lemon zest

½ teaspoon cinnamon

½ teaspoon sea salt

1 pound ground lamb

2 tablespoons solid cooking fat

½ cup Bone Broth (page 34)

4 cups baby spinach leaves

½ lemon, juiced
  (about 1 tablespoon)

1 Combine the olives, garlic, lemon zest, cinnamon, and salt in a bowl.

2 Add the lamb, mix thoroughly, and form into 1-inch meatballs.

3 Heat the cooking fat in a skillet on medium-high heat.

4 When the fat has melted and the pan is hot, cook the meatballs for 5 minutes, turning periodically to get all sides browned. Add the bone broth and cover, cooking for another 5 to 6 minutes until the meatballs are cooked throughout. Turn off the heat, add the spinach and stir until wilted.

5 Drizzle with lemon juice and serve.

Storage: Keeps in the refrigerator for several days.

Serving Suggestions: Puréed Parsnips (page 196), Mashed Sweet Potatoes (page 192)

ROSEMARY SHREDDED BEEF SKILLET

TOOLS | TIME | YIELD | DIFFICULTY

3-4

45 MINUTES | SERVINGS | ●●○○

3 tablespoons solid cooking fat

3 medium sweet potatoes, peeled and chopped into 1-inch cubes (about 4 cups)

½ yellow onion, chopped

2 cups chopped zucchini squash

4 cloves garlic, minced

2 tablespoons minced fresh rosemary

½ teaspoon sea salt

2 cups Shredded Roast Beef (page 261)

1 Heat 2 tablespoons of the cooking fat in the bottom of a large cast-iron pan or skillet on medium heat.

2 When the fat has melted and the pan is hot, add the sweet potatoes and cook, stirring, for 10 minutes, or until they are slightly soft, but not all the way cooked. Add the onion and cook for another 5 minutes, then add the zucchini, garlic, rosemary, and salt, stirring. Cook for 10 more minutes.

3 Add the shredded beef and the rest of the cooking fat. Cook for another few minutes, until the beef is heated through and all of the vegetables are soft.

Variation: Try using hard winter squash (like butternut or acorn) instead of the sweet potato.

Storage: Keeps in the refrigerator for several days.

Serving Suggestions: Sautéed Market Greens (page 183), Seared Broccolini with Coconut-Basil Pesto (page 204)

LAMB CHOPS WITH
ROSEMARY-PLUM SAUCE

TOOLS	TIME	YIELD	DIFFICULTY
	45 MINUTES	**4-6** SERVINGS	●●●○

2 tablespoons solid cooking fat

½ onion, chopped

2 cloves garlic, minced

3 firm plums, chopped into
2-inch pieces (about 1 ½ cups)

1 tablespoon minced rosemary

¼ teaspoon sea salt

2 pounds lamb rib chops

1 Heat 1 tablespoon of the cooking fat in a saucepan on medium heat. When the fat has melted and the pan is hot, add the onion and cook for about 5 minutes. Add the garlic and cook for another minute, stirring. Add one plum, and cook for about 10 minutes, stirring, until soft. Turn off the heat.

2 Transfer the mixture to a blender and purée it. Add the mixture back to the pot, along with the remaining chopped plums, rosemary and half of the salt. Turn the heat to medium and cook for 10 more minutes, or until the sauce has thickened and the plums are soft.

3 Sprinkle the remaining salt on the lamb chops, and heat the remaining cooking fat in a skillet on high heat. Sauté the lamb chops 5 to 8 minutes per side, or until desired doneness is reached.

4 Serve the chops with plum sauce drizzled over the top.

Storage: Keeps in the refrigerator for several days.

Serving Suggestions: Cucumber-Mint Salad (page 141), Radish and Jicama Tabbouli (page 142), Puréed Parsnips (page 196)

"SPAGHETTI" AND MEATBALLS

TOOLS **TIME** 30 MINUTES **YIELD** 4 SERVINGS **DIFFICULTY** ●●●○

2 pounds grass-fed ground beef

1 tablespoon minced fresh rosemary

1 tablespoon minced fresh thyme

1 tablespoon minced fresh sage

1 teaspoon sea salt

2 tablespoons solid cooking fat

1 recipe Nomato Sauce (page 135)

4 zucchini, cut into noodles with a mandoline or spiralizer

Fresh basil, for garnish

Zest of 1 lemon, for garnish

1 In a large bowl, combine the ground beef, fresh herbs, and salt.

2 Using your hands, form into large, 2- to 3-inch meatballs.

3 Heat 1 tablespoon of the cooking fat in a skillet on medium heat. Add the meatballs and brown well on all sides. Add the Nomato Sauce, cover and turn down to a simmer. Cook for another 10 to 15 minutes, or until the meatballs are cooked throughout.

4 Meanwhile, heat the remaining cooking fat in the bottom of another skillet or a wok. When the fat has melted and the pan is hot, add the zucchini noodles and cook, tossing them gently, until they soften (about 5 minutes).

5 Serve a plate of zucchini noodles, meatballs, and sauce garnished with the chopped basil and lemon zest.

Variation: Feel free to use any kind of ground meat for this recipe, or a combination thereof. You can also replace the zucchini noodles with cooked spaghetti squash.

Storage: Keeps in the refrigerator for several days.

Serving Suggestions: Emerald Kale Salad (page 138), Brussels Sprouts with Crispy Bacon (page 191), Sautéed Market Greens (page 183)

SWEET TREATS

CINNAMON-GINGER BAKED PEARS

TOOLS | TIME | YIELD | DIFFICULTY

1 HOUR

4
SERVINGS

●●○○

2 tablespoons Coconut
  Concentrate (page 45)*
2 firm pears, halved and cored
1 tablespoon coconut oil, melted
½ lemon, juiced
  (about 1 tablespoon)
⅛ teaspoon cinnamon
⅛ teaspoon ginger
Pinch of sea salt

1 Preheat the oven to 350 degrees F.

2 Brush the pear halves generously with coconut oil and lemon juice. Mix the cinnamon, ginger, and salt in a small bowl and sprinkle evenly over the pears.

3 Place the pears cut side up in a baking dish and bake for 30 minutes, or until soft. Remove from the oven and let cool for a few minutes.

4 Drizzle with coconut concentrate and serve immediately.

*Note: In order to measure the coconut concentrate, it is best to soften it in a warm water bath before use as it is solid at room temperature.

Variation: Feel free to use apples for this recipe, but they may take a bit longer to bake.

Storage: Keeps in the refrigerator for several days.

APPLE-SPICE TEA COOKIES

TOOLS	TIME	YIELD	DIFFICULTY
	45 MINUTES	**8** COOKIES	●●○○

1 cup fine shredded coconut
   flakes (unsweetened)

2 tablespoons coconut flour

1 apple, peeled, cored, and
   roughly chopped

8 dates, pitted

2 tablespoons coconut oil

¼ teaspoon cinnamon

Pinch of sea salt

1 Preheat the oven to 325 degrees F.

2 Place all ingredients in a food processor and mix until a thick paste forms. Form into 8 round, flat cookies and place on a baking sheet greased with a little coconut oil.

3 Bake for 15 minutes, or until barely golden. The cookies will still be a little soft; let cool completely before serving.

Variation: Feel free to use pears for this recipe. You can also use dried figs instead of dates for a less sweet cookie.

Storage: Keeps in the refrigerator for a week. Also freezes well.

CHERRY-LIME POPSICLES

TOOLS   TIME   YIELD   DIFFICULTY

30 MINUTES
SET 3 HOURS

6
POPSICLES

3 cups frozen pitted cherries (unsweetened)

½ cup freshly squeezed lime juice (about 12 limes)

½ teaspoon lime zest

¼ teaspoon sea salt

1 Pour the cherries into a shallow dish or bowl and allow them to partially thaw. Put the cherries, lime juice, zest, and salt in a blender and blend until smooth.

2 Pour the mixture into popsicle molds. Freeze completely and serve.

Storage: Keeps in the freezer for a month.

Variation: Substitute frozen berries or pineapple for the cherries.

MANGO-COCONUT POPSICLES

TOOLS   TIME   YIELD   DIFFICULTY

30 MINUTES
SET 3 HOURS

6
POPSICLES

3 cups frozen mango

½ cup coconut water

½ teaspoon lemon zest

¼ teaspoon sea salt

1 Put the mango into a shallow dish or bowl and allow them to partially thaw. Put the mango, coconut water, zest, and salt into a blender and blend until smooth.

2 Pour the mixture into popsicle molds. Freeze completely and serve.

Storage: Keeps in the freezer for a month.

COCONUT CREAM BOWL

TOOLS   TIME   YIELD   DIFFICULTY

15 MINUTES   **4** SERVINGS

½ cup Coconut Concentrate (page 45)*

½ cup filtered water

¼ cup honey

¼ teaspoon sea salt

¼ cup raspberries

½ cup strawberries, stemmed and halved

¼ cup kiwi fruit, peeled, halved, and cut into thin slices

Pinch of cinnamon

1 Place the coconut concentrate, water, honey, and salt in a blender and blend for a few seconds, or until thoroughly incorporated. If mixture is too thick, add more water a tablespoon at a time until desired consistency is reached.

2 Divide the mixture into four cups or bowls and top with the fresh fruit. Add a dusting of cinnamon to each, and serve immediately.

*Note: In order to measure the coconut concentrate, it is best to soften it in a warm water bath before use as it is solid at room temperature.

Variation: Feel free to switch up the fruit and spices—mango and lime zest would be nice, as would pomegranate seeds or blackberries.

MACAROONS

TOOLS	TIME	YIELD	DIFFICULTY
	30 MINUTES	12 MACAROONS	●●○○

2 cups plus 2 tablespoons unsweetened coconut flakes

1 ½ cups dates, pitted and soaked in warm water for 5 minutes

¼ teaspoon alcohol-free vanilla extract (optional)

¼ teaspoon sea salt

1 Preheat the oven to 325 degrees F.

2 Place the 2 cups of coconut flakes, dates, vanilla (if using), and sea salt in a food processor and process until thick and sticky.

3 Place the remaining coconut flakes on a small plate. Form the date mixture into little balls, rolling in coconut flakes for decoration.

4 Place on a greased cookie sheet and bake for 12 to 15 minutes, or until barely golden.

Lemon Variation: Add 1 tablespoon lemon juice and 1 teaspoon lemon zest to the coconut and date mixture.

Blueberry Variation: Add 3/4 cup frozen or fresh blueberries to the coconut and date mixture.

Storage: Keeps in the refrigerator for a week. Also freezes well.

RASPBERRY-COCONUT "CHEESECAKE"

TOOLS   TIME   YIELD   DIFFICULTY

12

1 HOUR +
24 HRS TO SET

SERVINGS

●●●●

Crust:

3 cups dates, pitted and soaked for 5 minutes in warm water

1 cup coconut oil, melted

⅓ cup coconut flour

⅓ cup fine shredded coconut flakes (unsweetened)

⅛ teaspoon salt

Filling:

1 ½ cups Coconut Concentrate (page 45)

1 ½ cups whipped honey

1 cup coconut oil, melted

4 cups frozen raspberries

6 tablespoons tapioca starch

1 ½ teaspoons vanilla extract (optional)

¼ teaspoon sea salt

Thick, unsweetened coconut flakes, for garnish

Fresh raspberries, for garnish

1 Preheat the oven to 325 degrees F.

2 To prepare the crust, strain the dates (discard the water) and place them in a food processor or high-powered blender with the melted coconut oil. Blend for 30 seconds or so until a chunky paste forms. Note: if you are using a standard blender, you may have to stop and scrape the sides, and the oil may not completely mix with the dates, but the crust will still turn out fine.

3 Combine the coconut flour, shredded coconut, and salt in a bowl. Add the date paste and mix thoroughly. Place the mixture in the bottom of an 8-inch springform pan, pressing it down evenly. Use a small spatula to clean up the top edge around the sides of the pan, where the filling will meet the crust. Bake for 30 to 35 minutes, until the crust browns and hardens a little bit. The texture will still be soft until it finishes cooling. Set aside while you make the filling.

4 Soften the coconut concentrate and honey by placing them in a warm water bath for a few minutes.

5 To make the filling, combine the coconut concentrate, honey, coconut oil, and frozen raspberries in a saucepan on low heat. Stir until the raspberries are no longer frozen and the mixture is warm, about 5 minutes. Transfer to a blender and add the tapioca starch, vanilla extract, and salt. Blend on high for about a minute, until completely mixed. Pour carefully on top of the crust.

6 Set in the refrigerator undisturbed for at least 12 hours to allow the cake to cool and completely solidify. When it is ready, carefully remove the sides of the springform pan.

7 Decorate the top of the cake with thick-flake coconut chips and fresh raspberries.

Note: For best results, use a honey that is solid at room temperature, like a whipped product. Make sure you use Coconut Concentrate (page 45), which is not the same as the thick stuff at the top of a can of coconut milk! If you used the canned coconut milk, the cake will not set.

Variation: Substitute 3 cups of blueberries for the 4 cups raspberries; for a blueberry-lemon variation, add the juice and zest of 1 lemon.

Storage: Keeps for a week, tightly wrapped, in the refrigerator. Leftover slices can be frozen for later enjoyment!

APPLE-CRANBERRY CRUMBLE

TOOLS TIME YIELD DIFFICULTY

8

1 HOUR SERVINGS

Crumble:

1 ½ cups coconut oil, cold
1 cup coconut flour
1 cup arrowroot flour
1 cup coconut sugar
1 teaspoon cinnamon
¼ teaspoon sea salt
½ cup cold filtered water

Filling:

6 apples, chopped into 1 ½-inch
  pieces
1 cup unsweetened dried
  cranberries
¼ cup coconut oil, melted
1 lemon, juiced
  (about 2 tablespoons)
1 teaspoon cinnamon

1 Preheat the oven to 350 degrees F. If the coconut oil is not already cold, put it in the refrigerator for about 10 minutes to chill.

2 In a large bowl, combine the coconut flour, arrowroot flour, coconut sugar, cinnamon, and salt. Using a pastry cutter, cut in the coconut oil until you have pea-size lumps. Sprinkle in the cold water, and gently mix—you want the crumble topping to stay chunky and not turn into dough. Set aside.

3 In another large bowl, combine the apples, cranberries, coconut oil, lemon juice, and cinnamon. Mix until well combined. Place in a 9-by-13-inch baking dish and cover with the crumble topping.

4 Bake for 40 minutes, until lightly browned on top. Remove from the oven, let cool a little bit and serve warm.

Variation: Feel free to use pears instead of apples, or raisins instead of cranberries.

Storage: Keeps in the refrigerator for several days; also freezes well.

PEAR-CARAMEL PIE

TOOLS | TIME | YIELD | DIFFICULTY

1 HOUR +
30 MINUTES

6
SERVINGS

● ● ● ●

Crust:

1 cup coconut flour

1 cup arrowroot flour

¼ teaspoon sea salt

¾ cup coconut oil, cold

½ cup cold filtered water

1 tablespoon coconut oil, melted

Filling:

3 tablespoons coconut oil

¼ cup coconut sugar

1 teaspoon cinnamon

½ teaspoon sea salt

1 teaspoon alcohol-free vanilla
   (optional)

4 firm pears

1 Preheat the oven to 325 degrees F. If the coconut oil is not already cold, put it in the refrigerator for about 10 minutes to chill.

2 Halve and core all of the pears, setting one aside and slicing the rest into thin, 1/4-inch slices.

3 In a bowl, combine the coconut flour, arrowroot flour, and salt. Using a pastry cutter, cut in the coconut oil until you have pea-size lumps. Add the cold water and mix. It will still be crumbly–not like regular dough! Don't over mix.

4 Place the mixture into a deep 9-inch pie dish. Using your fingers, spread it evenly across the bottom and up the sides. Prick some holes in the bottom of the crust with a fork, then brush the crust with the melted coconut oil. Bake for 15 minutes, until the crust browns. The texture will be soft as it finishes cooling. Set aside while you make the filling.

5 Heat the 3 tablespoons coconut oil and sugar for the filling in a medium saucepan. Cook for about 10 minutes, stirring until the sugar is caramelized and golden brown (don't be alarmed if it separates from the oil–this is normal). Pour the mixture into a bowl to cool a little bit before placing into a blender with the cinnamon, salt, vanilla (if using), and the pear that was cored but left unsliced. Blend on high until thoroughly mixed. Place the caramel sauce in a bowl and set aside.

6 Increase the oven temperature to 350 degrees F. Arrange the pear slices in a pinwheel, overlapping them, on top of the baked crust. Pour the caramel sauce evenly over the top; bake for 35 minutes, or until the crust is golden brown and the sauce is bubbling. Let cool for a few minutes and serve warm.

Variation: Feel free to use apples instead of pears here, although they may take longer to bake. You may also slice the fruit into chunks instead of making the pinwheel design.

Storage: Keeps in the refrigerator for several days; also freezes well.

ONLINE RESOURCES

autoimmune-paleo.com – My website, where I share recipes as well as articles about diet and autoimmunity.

balancedbites.com – A great resource by Diane Sanfilippo, author of *Practical Paleo*. Lots of information for those looking into ancestral nutrition or Paleo, with great ideas and recipes.

chriskresser.com – One of the best sources for scientific information about ancestral nutrition.

terrywahls.com – A resource for information on multiple sclerosis and diet by Terry Wahls, MD, who has put her own disease into remission using similar principles.

thepaleomom.com – The website of Sarah Ballantyne, PhD, author of *The Paleo Approach* and *The Paleo Approach Cookbook*. Her site is the best resource on the internet for information about the Autoimmune Protocol—It also contains many wonderful recipes.

whole9life.com - A great resource for those looking to try the autoimmune protocol in conjunction with Whole 30, a month-long clean eating challenge lead by Dallas and Melissa Hartwig.

Finding A Practitioner

functionalmedicine.org – The website of the Institute for Functional Medicine, where you can find a doctor who specializes in the functional treatment of autoimmune disease.

paleophysiciansnetwork.com – A website that helps you find a doctor who uses Paleo principles in their practice.

primaldocs.com – A resource to find a doctor or health care practitioner who uses an ancestral approach to health and nutrition.

thyroidconnections.com – A website that helps you find a practitioner who is trained by Dr. Datis Kharrazian to treat autoimmune thyroid disease.

Hashimoto's Disease

facebook.com/groups/EPDiet411/ - A wonderful support group for those interested in the elimination/provocation diet run by Kirsten Liston.

hashimotoshealing.com – Excellent information on the functional treatment of Hashimoto's disease by Marc Ryan, LaC.

stopthethyroidmadness.com – A great resource for thyroid patients to learn more about treatment options.

thyroidbook.com – Dr. Datis Kharrazian's website, which has information about functional medicine and Hashimoto's disease.

Autoimmune Protocol Patient Blogs

acleanplate.com – Written by Christina Feindel, a patient advocate with Hashimoto's—this site has lots of great allergen-free recipes.

alt-ternativeautoimmune.com – A blog by Angie Alt, who has used the protocol to heal from multiple autoimmune diseases. Angie shares recipes as well as the emotional side of healing from autoimmunity.

nutrisclerosis.com – An inspiring blog about the Autoimmune Protocol written by a woman with multiple sclerosis, Whitney Gray.

paleoparents.com – An excellent blog about Paleo, parenting, and the Autoimmune Protocol, written by Stacy Toth and Matthew McCarry.

phoenixhelix.com – A blog written by Eileen Laird, a woman who has used the protocol to heal her Rheumatoid Arthritis.

somerealitybites.com - A blog about living, learning, and thriving with Hashimoto's disease written by Susan Vennerholm.

Sourcing Food

autoimmune-paleo.com/amazon – My Amazon.com store with links to all of the pantry items referenced in the book.

azurestandard.com – Online co-op taking orders in bulk for organic food products and pastured meats.

eatwild.org – Use their search tool to connect with farmers in your area who sell quality meat or produce.

ewg.org/foodnews – "Dirty dozen" guide to which fruits and vegetables contain the highest amounts of pesticides.

grasslandbeef.com – An online retailer of high-quality pastured meat products.

localharvest.org – A website that can help you locate a farmer's market near you.

tropicaltraditions.com – An online retailer of organic coconut products as well as other staples and pastured meats.

Bone Broth

balancedbites.com/2011/04/easy-recipe-mineral-rich-bone-broth.html

westonaprice.org/food-features/broth-is-beautiful

Fermented Beverages

culturesforhealth.com

kombuchakamp.com

Fermented Vegetables

culturesforhealth.com

wildfermentation.com

Books For Continuing Education

Digestive Health with Real Food: A Practical Guide to an Anti-Inflammatory, Nutrient-Dense Diet for IBS and Other Digestive Issues, by Aglaee Jacob

It Starts With Food: Discover the Whole30 and Change Your Life in Unexpected Ways by Dallas and Melissa Hartwig

Hashimoto's Thyroiditis: Lifestyle Interventions for Treating the Root Cause, by Izabella Wentz

Practical Paleo: A Customized Approach to Health and a Whole-Foods Lifestyle, by Diane Sanfilippo

The Autoimmune Paleo Breakthrough: A Revolutionary Protocol to Rapidly Decrease Inflammation and Balance Your Immune System, by Anne Angelone

The Hidden Plague: A Field Guide For Surviving and Overcoming Hidradenitis Suppurativa, by Tara Grant

The Paleo Approach: Reverse Autoimmune Disease, Heal Your Body, by Sarah Ballantyne

The Paleo Approach Cookbook: A Detailed Guide to Heal Your Body and Nourish Your Soul, by Sarah Ballantyne

The Paleo Solution: The Original Human Diet, by Robb Wolf

Why Do I Still Have Thyroid Symptoms When My Lab Tests Are Normal: A Revolutionary Breakthrough in Understanding Hashimoto's Disease and Hypothyroidism, By Datis Kharrazian

Why Isn't My Brain Working: A Revolutionary Understanding of Brain Decline and Effective Strategies to Recover Your Brain's Health by Datis Kharrazian

Conversion Table:

Liquid

1 teaspoon = 5 mL
1 tablespoon = 15 mL
1 ounce = 30 mL
1/4 cup (2 oz) = 60 mL
1/3 cup = 80 mL
1/2 (4 oz) cup = 120 mL
3/4 cup (6 oz) = 180 mL
1 cup (8 oz) = 240 mL
1 quart = 950mL
1 gallon = 3.8L

Length

1/2 inch = 13mm
1 inch = 2.5 cm

Temperature

250 degrees F = 130 degrees C
300 degrees F = 150 degrees C
350 degrees F = 177 degrees C
400 degrees F = 200degrees C
450 degrees F = 230 degrees C
500 degrees F = 260 degrees C

Weight

1 ounce = 28g
1/4 pound (4 ounces) = 113g
1/2 pound (8 ounces) = 230g
3/4 pound (12 ounces) = 340g
1 pound (16 ounces) = 450g
2 pounds (32 oundes) = 900g

ABOUT THE AUTHOR

Mickey Trescott lives in Seattle, Washington, with her crafty husband and a rather pudgy Russian Blue cat. She practices nutritional therapy and cooks privately for local families in addition to blogging and obsessively knitting socks in her spare time. After recovering from her own struggle with both Celiac and Hashimoto's disease, adrenal fatigue, and multiple vitamin deficiencies, Mickey started to blog about her experiences at autoimmune-paleo.com. Her hope is to give others on a similar path a resource to find information—and to help them realize that they are not alone in their struggles. She also aims to provide a supportive environment for those seeking better health in the face of autoimmunity.

ABOUT THE PHOTOGRAPHER

Hailing from the Pacific Northwest, Kyle Johnson creates images that are intriguing and classically executed. Whether it's portrait or travel work, Kyle's aesthetic pairs textured natural settings with a distinct photographic perspective. He has shot for publications like *The New York Times Magazine, Wallpaper*, Sunset, Kinfolk, Popular Mechanics,* and more.

GRATITUDE

Thank you to all who have supported me in the journey of writing my first cookbook! It has been an incredible experience, and I would not have been able to do it without the support of many people.

Thank you to my friends, family, and blog readers who supported the crowd-funding campaign to produce this book—I am grateful for your contributions!

Thank you Kim Myers for stepping in at the last minute and helping to create a gorgeous cover image, and to Mary Cloos for the last-minute proof-read.

Thank you to Edward and Nancy at Star Print Brokers, for graciously answering all of my questions and making self-publishing a breeze. Thank you to Lisa and Jeffrey, for your patience and support through this process.

Thank you to Devyn Perez, Eric Elliott, Jane Thomas, Katie Sullivan, Felix Madrid, Rob Miller, Susan Vennerholm, Melanie Penney, and Jenny Littlefield for helping test recipes and assisting me on photo-shoot days.

Thank you to Crown S. Ranch and Olsen Farms for sustainably raising the quality meat I used to develop my recipes.

Thank you to Kyle Johnson, Brenna Rose Miller, and Chris Black, for being an incredible team and enabling me to produce such a high-quality book.

Thank you to my parents, Rose and Brian, for their endless love and support and for always encouraging me to follow my dreams.

Lastly, thank you to my husband Noah, who encouraged me to write this book in the first place – I am sorry you didn't know what you were getting yourself into! (but I hope the food was worth it . . .)

RECIPE INDEX

INDEX

REFERENCES

1. "Autoimmune Statistics," American Autoimmune Related Diseases Association, Inc, accessed September 15, 2013, http://www.aarda.org/autoimmune-information/autoimmune-statistics.

2. Sarah Ballantyne, *The Paleo Approach: Reverse Autoimmune Disease, Heal Your Body* (Las Vegas: Victory Belt, 2013), 53-57

3. Datis Kharrazian, *Why Do I Still Have Thyroid Symptoms? When My Lab Tests Are Normal: A Revolutionary Breakthrough in Understanding Hashimoto's Disease and Hypothyroidism* (Carlsbad: Elephant Press, 2010), 123-124

4. Robb Wolf, *The Paleo Solution: The Original Human Diet* (Las Vegas: Victory Belt, 2010), 201

5. Robb Wolf, *The Paleo Solution: The Original Human Diet* (Las Vegas: Victory Belt, 2010), 197-210

6. Sarah Ballantyne, *The Paleo Approach: Reverse Autoimmune Disease, Heal Your Body* (Las Vegas: Victory Belt, 2013), 185-186

7. Sarah Ballantyne, *The Paleo Approach: Reverse Autoimmune Disease, Heal Your Body* (Las Vegas: Victory Belt, 2013), 185-235

8. Sarah Ballantyne, *The Paleo Approach: Reverse Autoimmune Disease, Heal Your Body* (Las Vegas: Victory Belt, 2013), 53-57

9. Datis Kharrazian, *Why Do I Still Have Thyroid Symptoms? When My Lab Tests Are Normal: A Revolutionary Breakthrough in Understanding Hashimoto's Disease and Hypothyroidism* (Carlsbad: Elephant Press, 2010), 123

10. Aglaee Jacob, *Digestive Health with REAL Food: A Practical Guide to an Anti-Inflammatory, Nutrient Dense Diet for IBS and Other Digestive Issues* (Bend: Paleo Media group, 2013), 16-18

11. Sarah Ballantyne, *The Paleo Approach: Reverse Autoimmune Disease, Heal Your Body* (Las Vegas: Victory Belt, 2013), 264

12. Elson M. Haas, *Staying Healthy With Nutrition, The Complete Guide to Diet and Nutritional Medicine* (New York: Ten Speed Press, 2006), 83-248